1

Arthritis Treatments That Work

by Anthony di Fabio

Published under the name of *The Art of Getting Well* in June 10, 1988 Copyriight by the Arthritis Trust of America a non-profit, tax-exempt charity foundation, dedicated for research and communication about arthritis.

Publisher certifies that this is an independent news report made as accurately as possible, and further certifies that no drug company, medical doctor, or medically related institution has any financial interest in the sale and proceeds of this publication or the medicines recommended. Publisher further advises that all treatment should be through a licensed physician, and that we cannot be responsible for mal-application or mis-application or inappropriate treatment of any kind. Voluntary contributions to the tax-exempt, charitable The Roger Wyburn-Mason and Jack M. Blount Foundation for the Eradication of Rheumatoid Disease, Inc.(The Arthritis Trust of America/The Rheumatoid Disease Foundation), 7111 Sweetgum Road, Fairview, TN 37062-9384 will be used for the purpose of furthering research and education.

Chapter I
Can Rheumatoid Arthritis Be Cured?

You've been told that Rheumatoid Arthritis is not curable. That is false!

If the statement disturbs you, do not read further. Do not learn how thousands are finding relief and even wellness. Do not give up your aspirin, your non-steroidal anti-inflammatories. Do not quit your visits to your favorite rheumatologist. Do not stop paying for ineffective and damaging gold, penicillamine, methotrexate and cortisone.

If you are one of those who are filled with pain day and night, and want relief — if you are a person who views the future as a cripple with constantly decreasing abilities and want to stop the crippling — if you're a man or woman or child who lives pain-free but minutes and then only at the will of a drug, a doctor, a drug store, and by courtesy of a fat pocketbook — but especially if you are a person who wants relief from this century's-long scourge — you'll want to absorb this book in it's entirety, you'll want to read further!

In 1980s thirteen million Americans suffered from so-called incurable Rheumatoid Diseases. Three million were restricted in their daily activities. Seven hundred thousand could not do useful work, keep house, attend school or enjoy recreational activities. One out of three of us either had a form of the disease or will display some symptoms of arthritis — if we live long enough!

Tens of millions of Americans suffer from Osteoarthritis and Gouty Arthritis. Some predict that almost everyone will develop some form of Arthritis if he/she lives long enough.

The Rheumatoid Disease Foundation takes the stand that there is no difference between so-called "Adult Rheumatoid Arthritis" and "Juvenile Rheumatoid Arthritis". Both age groups respond to the treatments to be described.

If left untreated, Rheumatoid Arthritis and other forms of Rheumatoid Diseases can become progressively worse, eventually leading to painful crippling, but this is particularly true of Rheumatoid Arthritis, which can and will destroy the joints unless effective treatment is administered in time.

Those who tell you that nothing much can be done for Arthritis are only fooling themselves and you. A great deal can be done, as you will learn — and crippling is not inevitable.

Most arthritis victims suffer pain, but we will show several ways that pain can be controlled and possibly alleviated entirely.

The sooner you begin treatment for Arthritis, the more probability of having success in halting its progress and perhaps cleaning up or reversing damage that has begun -- providing your treatments are the correct ones for you!

Then there are those who tell you that, "Once you have Arthritis, chances are great that you're stuck with it for life," and "You should learn to adjust to it, for better or worse." "Don't look for a cure or relief, but learn to control your symptoms" — those people are telling you to give up, to permit the crippling to go on, to get yourself ready for a life of total misery and acceptance of your fate.

Those same advisors are also ignorant of any other means of helping you, or they would not be giving you such advice. They have given up. You don't need to give up too!

You must make a choice. Do you wish to follow such "establishment medicine" practices? Or do you wish to fight for your survival and some of the good things in life, including the right to live unhindered from pain and crippling?

No pharmaceutical company is interested in curing or stopping the progress of our disease. They are interested in maintaining our dependency drug habits so that corporate stock owners and upper management can swell up their pocketbooks. Ideally, when a drug company can develop an exclusive, patented drug upon which arthritics must rely — as a drug addict must rely on habit-forming drugs — then the drug company is content. They are especially happy if the medicine relieves symptoms and forces us to spend more and more on the drug to simply maintain the appearances of wellness — and the disease rages onward!

Cortisone provides only symptomatic relief, as its sale and medicinal administration to arthritics illustrates very well. Cortisone provides temporary and spectacular pain relief and the glow of false wellness. We must take increasing quantities over time to achieve this effect at the level we received earlier. During that period our bodies produce less and less of it. Eventually, over time, we quit producing cortisol at all. (Hydrocortisone is closely related to cortisone.) Thereafter, without periodic cortisone purchased from a drug company, by doctor's prescription, we die.

This book may not restore your ability to produce your own cortisol, a substance similar to cortisone, and it may not restore your deformed joints, but read on. It may restore your hope in a livable future, a sense of adventure, and a faith that you've possibly buried beneath tons of pain and agony — perhaps wellness!

Treated by the hundreds of physicians who follow our treatment protocol properly, there are already tens of thousands of former arthritics — folks like you and me — who have found great relief, improvement and yes, even complete wellness.

I was an arthritic — perhaps just as you are now — but I am free of the horrible disease and I've been free for more than thirty years!.

I intend to convince you to take command of your life again, to learn for yourself ways and means of achieving wellness and again peace of mind. I will describe what you can do and I will recommend that you work with a caring physician. If necessary, you must search out and find a physician who is not bound by that ancient arrogance which prevents some physicians from learning further and the patient from achieving wellness.

Eighty percent of those who follow my directions will either be cured or improved immensely and the disease halted. If you are among those whose bodily functions (immunological system) have already been damaged by traditional treatments that use gold, penicillamine, methotrexate and long-term cortico-steroids, the news is still favorable and better than your present outlook. About 50% of this latter group get well or vastly improved, especially when they are willing and able to halt these destructive treatments for a few months prior to starting the one recommended herein. Usually after permitting bodily systems to recover throughout four months, the immunological system responds sufficiently to our treatment.

Traditional treatment can expect to achieve relief or the temporary appearance of wellness but 33% of the time.

The placebo effect — the percentage of patients who will improve (at least temporarily) no matter what the physician does — is about 33% for arthritics. It follows, therefore, that traditional treatments are not effective any better than chance alone, for which we pay out $15 billion a year.

The treatments described in this book are therefore at least 165% or better than traditional, accepted but ineffective treatments.

I have no vested interest in the sale of drugs, foods, medical treatments, vitamins and minerals, physicians or clinics. I work for a non-profit, charitable, tax-exempt foundation dedicated to solving the problems of Rheumatoid Disease by means of education and research. The profit, if any, on the sale of this book will go for education and research.

This book chiefly condenses The Rheumatoid Disease Foundation/The Arthritis Trust of America findings of the past five years and while it's recommendations are in advance of anything else written on arthritis, it will not be the last and final word. Scientific progress means change. Solving Rheumatoid Arthritis and related diseases means changing both the modalities of present-day treatment and our own attitudes toward it. At the end of this book we will present everything we've learned about Rheumatoid Disease causations since 1982!

To your family doctor, we say: Our treatment protocol has never been considered for use against Rheumatoid Arthritis because the various rheumatologists and arthritis associations have not investigated Professor Roger Wyburn-Mason's brilliant scientific work, published since 1964, that led to the treatment to be described.

You must decide if the prescriptions that follow are harmful to your patient. If not, is the cost involved worth a trial, considering the hopeless and insidious nature of the disease?

Many cooperating physicians, and their patients, use and have used the protocol developed by this Rheumatoid Disease Foundation — more than two hundred physicians, tens of thousands of patients, represented in seventeen (1999) countries.

To you, the Rheumatoid Arthritis victim, we say that what follows covers more than our own suggestion for wellness — or at least in improving the quality of your life — more will be described than simply the Foundation Treatment Protocol. Many of the suggested treatments are recommended by the writer because of his personal experiences, although it is true that some chapters came into being because of successes reported by other patients or physicians who tried the treatments described therein.

Rheumatoid Disease Foundation referral physicians contributed greatly through their clinical experiences. In particular, thanks to John Baron, D.O., Gus Prosch, Jr., M.D. and Tony Chapdelaine, M.D., MPH for their assistance and advice (which I did not always take). Where errors exist, and wrong interpretations of medical facts, the author, solely, is to blame.

Finally, if you're in a hurry, go to the last part of this book where you'll find a summary on those areas of your life that you should explore to learn the causation, and to eliminate the causation of your painful malady.

The Rheumatoid Disease Foundation cannot, of course, be responsible for mal-application, mis-application, or inappropriate treatment of any kind, and suggest strongly that treatment, if possible, be through your family physician.

I pray that you will be among those who read and

follow recommendations where appropriate. Our common goal?

To rid the earth of this terrible, crippling plague, called Arthritis! Cordially,

Anthony di Fabio

Chapter II
You Must Judge

An arthritic needs no description of his disease's progress, nor his painful symptoms that distort the joints into such grotesque forms, leading inevitably to surgery and certain crippling. But even the arthritic needs to be able to differentiate those arthritic symptoms that represent an on-going disease process — active disease — as compared to the damage that has already been done or will be done.

Symptoms of an active, on-going disease process are usually tissue swelling (edema), warm or hot joints (pyrexia), lethargy and depression, and, most importantly, an <u>increasing</u> number of painful joints.

When we state that we can stop the progress of Rheumatoid Disease for 80% of the victims who properly use our treatment protocol, we speak specifically of halting and reducing tissue swelling, restoring joints and tissues to normal temperature and stopping the <u>increase</u> in the number of joints that become affected and painful. Depression and lethargy may also stop, and will certainly do so with further related treatments of a different nature, as with the pain that might remain in joints after treatment. It is totally possible, and has happened frequently, that no related treatments will be required, but don't count on a simple approach to clear up everything at once. More will be explained on this later.

So what about the already crippled-up joints, and residual pain and lethargy and depression that might remain?

The on-going disease process reflects itself through the swelling (edema) and heat (pyrexia), and just as these are symptomatic processes — evidence that something is wrong — the <u>result</u> of all those biochemical processes shows up as damaged, painful joints, lethargy and depression.

There is more complexity, but we shall unwind a lot of it. For now, remember the term "free-radical damage". For the purpose of this book, we shall define "free-radical damage" as secondary damage that accompanies Rheumatoid Disease while it is active or "flared up". This definition is not scientifically accurate or complete, but neither is this a textbook of science.

Even if you are an arthritic, you have probably been viewing your symptoms in a way that includes <u>all</u> characteristics of the disease — the "on-going process" characteristics and the "secondary damage" characteristics caused by the "on-going process" — as a complete package. How many times have you seen or heard the comment, "Oh, that's Rheumatoid Disease" when speaking of a crippled joint?

No!

The crippled joint is <u>not</u> the disease!

The crippled joint is a <u>result</u> of the disease!

When our treatment is used, and when it is effective, the symptoms of swelling and heated joints disappear, and the symptoms of joint pain may disappear, as may the symptoms of lethargy and depression. Most certainly other treatments to be described will probably rid one of joint pains and lethargy and depression unless irreversible damage is involved, such as permanently deformed joints. I have two small fingers with permanently deformed joints, for example.

I am not interested in convincing you on the emotional level of case histories. You have probably tried many other treatments that have not worked, and you will not be fearful of trying one more. You, like me, are probably tired of reading case histories of alleged success. Our treatment either works on you, or doesn't work at all. You and I care less about whether it worked on others, until we solve our own problem.

Like you, I was skeptical and even scoffed — but I tried this recommended treatment, for lack of anything better. Even my family doctor scoffed, saying, "Look, it won't help, but it can't harm you, so go ahead and try if you wish," and with that he approved of my taking two prescriptions sent to me by Dr. Blount and that started me on the path to wellness.

The truth is that no number of hearsay statements from and about successful patients will answer your big question. Since the treatment is safe — or at least extremely safe when compared against traditional treatments — your only question is, "will it be effective for me?" There is no way to answer such a question without giving our treatment protocols a fair trial — and only you will know whether or not you have tried honestly and fairly.

Be forewarned that many of the treatment methods to be described for you are not accepted treatments. Some related treatments to be described and which have also proved effective are being persecuted by unknowledgeable state medical boards and duped district attorneys in some states. While this blind rejection is not true of everything to be described, by being forewarned you will be able to better cope with scoffers and authoritarian figures who feel their control — and income — slipping away.

If Authorities knew the correct treatment, they would already be applying it, wouldn't they?

So don't be embarrassed if some would-be larger than life Authority denounces what is said herein, or argues against your trial of various treatments. Progress in medicine has always been thusly hindered, and your job as a patient is to separate the "It works for me!" from "It doesn't work for me!" And no number of Authorities can make it otherwise, and no one knows better than you whether or not the treatment fits one category or another. Our recommendations to get you well are for the most part safe, effective and cheap.

Remember this!

Not all the Authorities on earth and their scholastic, hob-goblined opinions can determine whether or not our treatment works for you!

You must judge for yourself

Chapter III
Rheumatoid Disease Newly Defined

The human body has a limited number of responses to various system disturbances. For example: Most everyone is familiar with headaches. While the pain of each headache may be very similar in nature each time experienced, the cause of each headache can vary considerably. Headaches might be caused by eyestrain, back or low musculature strain, biological disturbances of tissues or chemistry, suppressed emotion, and so on.

In other words, just because a person has a headache does not mean that the cause is self-evident, or necessarily simple, nor does the cause of <u>our</u> headache need to be related to the causes of our neighbors' or friends'.

While we are all genetically different, and have different bio-chemistries, our bodies seem to have limited ways of responding to varying stimuli.

It should be clear, therefore, that all symptoms described as "arthritic" are not symptoms that derive from the same cause. You already know about "Osteoarthritis", "Rheumatoid Arthritis" and "Gouty Arthritis", three of the most common with differing causes.

Rheumatoid Arthritis is characterized by specific symptoms: heated joints and body members, swelling, lethargy, depression and an increasing number of painful joints that eventually become damaged and crippled.

Since we look at only symptoms of a disease "in-process" we cannot say for sure that every time someone has these five characteristics he/she has the same disease as others.

When laboratory tests are used to narrow the causative agent(s), we are often led to costly tests that are virtually useless. The test that is labeled RF for "Rheumatoid Factor" is mis-labeled and probably does not test for Rheumatoid Arthritis at all. It tests a fraction of blood called "immunoglobulin" and is present in 70% of adults with Rheumatoid Arthritis. Some physicians have indicated that 25% of such tests are negative, when they should be positive, and 25% are positive when they should be negative. At best, the test measures probable existence of something akilter respecting our bodily systems, a fact we already know.

It is highly unlikely that any number of present-day laboratory tests (1987) can determine the existence or non-existence of Rheumatoid Disease. Often the physician makes such tests because it is the established and accepted thing to do, and because doing the established and accepted thing protects his/her medical insurance status. Neither of these reasons gets you properly diagnosed or well.

Sometimes these lab tests together with clinical experience and good judgment can deduce a set of possible causes that should be further explored by medical treatment trials. Those trials, even if unsuccessful, may lead to further educated guesses on the part of your physician that will eventually narrow causes down to one or more that are amendable to changes.

Your problem may be to find a physician who is willing to step outside of traditional treatment boundaries and to view you as a whole person, not just a statistic to warehouse in a small examination room pending arrival of his august presence, and there to be scrutinized but minutes, and thereafter to be given at relatively high cost a traditional, accepted, ineffective treatment.

Many in the medical community suspect a causative organism for Rheumatoid Disease such as bacteria, mycoplasma, yeast/fungus, protozoan, virus, cell wall deficient organism, or some combination or variation of these minute life forms.

They suspect that people are either born with a genetic susceptibility to these organisms or develop that genetic susceptibility later. "Genetic susceptibility" means an inborn sensitivity to the organism or toxin from the organism that causes our tissues to respond with the symptoms.

There is a high degree of suspicion that we have

developed, or are born with, an "allergy" to some organism that invades from outside our bodies. We develop "antibodies", fighters, for that "antigen", the invader, and there comes persistent warfare between our antibodies and the antigen that creates damage we see as the symptoms we call Rheumatoid Disease.

This suspicion may very well be true, and it serves as a good model, really the best predictor and hypothesis of the nature of the disease that we have to date. From a purely workable viewpoint, we can accept the model until developing a better one.

The antibody/antigen model serves to underline one very important aspect of Rheumatoid Disease. The disease is <u>not</u> localized in just one place! The disease is <u>systemic.</u> This means that even though you do not observe <u>symptoms</u> of the disease as raging onward in a particular portion of your body, the disease is there, believe me. It is just that, for the moment, you are manifesting the disease in a particular part of the body. These overt symptoms make you think the disease is localized to, say, a knee joint, or wrist joint. All of your attention is quite naturally on that spot, because that's where the pain, swelling and heat is for the moment.

If you accept the proposition that Rheumatoid Disease is systemic (throughout the body) in nature, it is clear that a treatment for purely local parts of the body is doomed to failure. Cortisone shots to relieve pain in a joint, for example, do not stop the process in either the joint or in the whole body, while they do help to erode the joint further.

There are two characteristics about Rheumatoid Disease to keep in mind. One is that Rheumatoid Disease symptoms may be the result of multiple causes. We see similarities between different people because our bodies are designed to respond in but limited ways. The second fact is that Rheumatoid Disease pervades the whole body, not just a local area.

Having stated the above two principles, we now mention possible "causes" of "arthritis". The symptoms of "arthritis" may be caused by any one or combination of the following:

1. Bacterial infections such as those resulting from invasion of gonococcal, tuberculosis, or pneumo- coccal germs.

2. Viruses, particularly RNA viral forms.

3. Yeast/fungus, particularly Candidas albicans.

4. Allergens, internal and/or external, as with foods, pollens, house dusts, invading organisms.

5. Weakened immunological system, caused by any of the above and including causation of improper nutrition, prolonged stress, etc.

6. Metabolic disturbances, as evident with Gout, Osteoarthritis, Osteoarthrosis.

7. Other unidentified and unnamed source causes.

All of the above, and perhaps more, may cause symptoms of Rheumatoid Arthritis. The portions of the body where the symptoms may appear are a multitude. To name a few, they are:

The arteries, as in periarteritis; bone, as in Paget's Disease, cysts and myelomas; brain and spinal cord, as displayed by tremors and seizures; bronchi, as with bronchitis, intrinsic asthma (as opposed to extrinsic; i.e. caused by an external allergen or external source); heart, as with dysrhythmias, myocardial disease, pericardial disease; cecum as with appendicitis, mesenteric adenitis; colon, as with ulcerative colitis; endocrine glands, as with thyroid, parathyroid, thymus, pituitary, adrenal glands; esophagus and stomach, producing atropic mucosa (pernicious anemia), webs; eyes, with iridocyclitis, exophthalmias; fascial planes, showing as bursitis; female genitals, for ovarian cysts, fibroids, salpingitis-sterility, tubal pregnancies; Hemopoetic, displaying as systemic lupus erythematosus, polycythemia, purpura; joints, as with arthritis; kidneys, pyelonephritis, calculi; liver, showing as hepatitis, cholangitis, gallbladder disease; lower small gut, displaying as regional enteritis, Crohn's Disease; lungs as with alveolitis; lymphatics (lymph system) for lymphomas, splenomegaly; meninges (covering around brain), producing headache, meningomas; muscles with myositis; nerves, trigeminal neuralgia; nose and throat, presenting as rhinitis, eustachian salpingitis, enlarged tonsils and adenoids; ovum, producing fetal deformities and abortions; pancreas with pancreatitis, maturity diabetes, noninsulin dependent diabetes; salivary and tear glands with SICCA syndrome; skin with psoriasis, alopecia, erythemas, urticaria; spine, degenerated discs and low back syndrome; tendons for tendonitis, ganglion; upper gut with coealic disease; and also functional central nervous system problems producing neuroses, psychosis and senility.

Since different parts of the body are involved, the symptoms presented to the physician are given different names, but many of those described can now be classified under one heading, that of "Rheumatoid Disease". This is the definition given by Professor Roger Wyburn-Mason, a brilliant research physician from England, now deceased, and whose treatment methods led to the first major improvements and cures.

There is a parallel, by analogy, between the old and

generally accepted view of "Rheumatoid Arthritis" and that cluster of diseases which your Foundation now titles "Rheumatoid Disease". Before the discovery of the tubercle baccilus, the germ that causes tuberculosis, there were about 150 differently named symptoms that patients presented to their doctor. The fact that each symptom was given a unique name sometimes appeased the patient, but certainly did not get them well.

After discovery of the tubercle bacillus all of those 100 or so names collapsed under the heading of

"TB of the bone", "TB of the lungs", "TB of the skin", and so on.

When I went to grade school (thirties) I was taught that everyone on earth was exposed to the TB germ, but that only a small number of people were genetically susceptible to the organism, thus coming down with TB. This may or may not have been true, but as a parallel analogy, and to produce a working hypothesis around which Rheumatoid Disease can be solved, the essentials appear to correspond. Rheumatoid Disease (hereafter often referred to as RD), has been given nearly a hundred different names; it now has but one, "Rheumatoid Disease" or "RD" and it seems to have a "genetic predisposition factor", i.e. people seem to be susceptible along genetic lines (inherited) to whatever causes the apparent antigen/antibody relationship.

All of the previously described diseases — and perhaps more — can occur in their pure forms, or in combinations with any of the other "labeled" diseases.

Naming a disease, as you know, does not get the person well any more so than treating a disease with the wrong medicine, or by the wrong treatment protocol. Most of the established and accepted treatments for RD are based on the presumption that there is something wrong with the immunological system, that portion of the body that fights off infection by recognizing a foreign protein as "not-me". If this presumption is wrong, there will be endless hours spent unraveling the complexity of the very obscure immunological system. There are, in fact, tons of books on this one subject, and it requires a highly trained specialist simply to understand details. It's sort of like being in the middle of a tangled woods and, rather than stepping out to understand the woods as a whole, one spends a lifetime learning about and studying each individual growth.

A perfect example of this "scientific" medical problem once existed with the lack of understanding of syphilis as a disease caused by an organism. Until the finding of the syphilis spirochete, the symptoms of syphilis presented to the research physician a perfect picture of an "auto-immune" disease; i.e., a disease wherein the immunological system fails to identify portions of the body as "self" and attacks the body as "non-self".

Now we know better that syphilis is a disease caused by an organism that comes from outside the body. It is not the consequence of a "failed" immunological system.

But consider the present day consequences to millions (and to organized society) if research physicians continued to insist that syphilis was a failure of the immunological system, an auto-immune disease, as all characteristics seemed to indicate before discovery of the spirochete! Tens of millions, perhaps hundreds of millions of dollars would have been expended in studying the immunological system, and thousands of dangerous drugs would have been invented and tried without success to modify or otherwise change a supposedly defective immunological system — to no avail!

But that situation indeed seems to prevail today in the attempt to understand and otherwise control arthritis!

We have no proof that those who pursue the small seedlings within the forest of the very complex immunological system are not correct. But they also have no proof that our hypothesis and treatment is not correct. We must be fair both ways, and perhaps both sides have a component of truth. You and I as arthritic victims care less what is believed or known, so long as we get well!

We shall take the assumption that there is a causative organism of origin or origins unknown. And from that presumption, simply as a working hypothesis, we expect to show 80% of those who try our treatment that they can indeed become greatly improved or cured completely. Other causations will be mentioned later.

Finally, to all of those who have written to the Foundation or will write to ask a certain question, we have the same advice. Since there are no definitive tests, if you wish to know if your particular symptoms will respond to the treatment to be described, you can only answer this yourself, by trying our recommendations fairly and honestly under supervision of a caring physician.

May both God and your own good sense go with you in the next adventure!

Chapter IV
Rheumatoid Disease Foundation Treatment Protocol

The Foundation's treatment protocol must be administered by a licensed physician, usually a Medical Doctor or Doctor of Osteopathy, or any physician who can prescribe the medicines that are to be recommended herein.

The physician must determine whether or not your body is capable of handling (metabolizing) the various medicines without danger, and whether or not interaction between various medicines that you may be taking will be safe.

Your physician must also make a determination that you do not suffer from neurological disease, such as Multiple Sclerosis (MS). If you have MS and should take some of the medicines described below, the progress of your MS may advance — which is obviously not what is desired.

In case that scares you, keep in mind that in the *Physician's Desk Reference* (a collection of drug companies' package inserts) the use of some of our recommended medicines already carries warning against use by Multiple Sclerosis victims, and that all ethical physicians know or seek to know the appplicable contents of the *Physician's Desk Reference* before prescribing for a patient.

Our recommended medicines used for the treatment and remission or cure of Rheumatoid Arthritis and related collagen diseases now called "Rheumatoid Diseases" are the following:

1. Metronidazole
2. Clotrimazole
3. Tinidazole
4. Nimorazole
5. Ornidazole
6. Allopurinol
7. Furazolidone
8. Diiodohydroxyquinon

9. Rifampin

10. Potassium Para Amino Benzoate

11. Copper Ions

Not all of the above medicines will work for everyone, and usually one must start with a commonly accepted medicine or combination of medicines, and make a trial, which will be described.

The brilliant English professor and physician, Roger Wyburn-Mason, M.D. Ph.D., discovered use of all of the above except Metronidazole, whose use for Rheumatoid Arthritis was discovered by the Mississippi physician, Jack M. Blount, Jr., M.D.; Diiodohydroxyquinon, whose use for these purposes was discovered by Robert Bingham, M.D. of California; and Seldon Nelson, D.O. of Michigan developed the use of Copper ions.

Our treatment protocol, which was designed by a committee of physicians under the umbrella of our referral physicians, and subsequently modified through clinical findings, follows:

If you are being treated with gold, penicillamine or methotrexate, then quit! Wait four months before taking our treatment, as your immunological system has already been so upset by these ineffective and often damaging treatments that your body probably will not respond well if at all to any of our medicines. DO NOT TAKE OUR TREATMENT AT THE SAME TIME YOU ARE TAKING GOLD, PENICILLAMINE OR METHOTREXATE. If you do you are simply laying the groundwork for maintaining the disease and related diseases at the same time you are using our recommended medicines to rid yourself of the disease. The reason is related to the weakening of your ability to fight diseases generally, and drug toxicity.

The effects of the use of corticosteroids (cortisone) are found at the microscopic level. It inhibits the early phenomena of the inflammatory process which includes swelling (edema), fibrin deposition (fibrin is responsible for blood clotting), capillary expansion (dilatation), migration of leukocytes (white blood cells) into the inflamed area, and phagocytic activity. Phagocytes search out and engulf and destroy foreign invaders. Cortisone also inhibits capillary proliferation, fibroblast proliferation, deposition of collagen and later scar tissue formation, all necessary for body growth and repair.

Cortisone has many well-known undesirable side-effects. It impairs wound healing and provides a predisposition to infection. It has major effects upon the monocyte/macrophage system, preventing release of Interleukin I, a substance that aids in fighting diseases. Large doses of corticosteroids results in a secondary problem of lymphopenia, a deficiency of lymphocytes in the blood. Monocytes are large mononuclear (one nucleus) leukocytes having more protoplasm (a thick viscous colloidal substance which constitutes the basis of all living activities) than a lymphocyte. Lymphocytes are lymph cells or white blood corpuscles without cytoplasmic granules (cytoplasmic protoplasm of a cell outside the nucleus). Macrophages have the ability to phagocytose (absorb and destroy) substances. Among our first line of defense against foreign invaders are to be found lymphocytes and macrophages.

If the language disturbs you, do not be concerned. Just remember that in people receiving cortisone, monocytes (large leukocytes that kill invaders) show an impaired ability to kill microorganisms. In the test tube there is an inhibition in the proliferation of T cells.

Helper and suppresser T cells in the blood stream have to be in the proper ratio, and they have a vital part in defending the body from foreign invaders. They also act in certain ways that causes macrophages to release the Interleukin 1. Interleukin 1 stimulates formation of Interleukin 2, the immediate stimulus for proliferation of T cells.

Corticosteroids (cortisone) lead to an increase in the number of polymorphonuclear leukocytes (white blood cells whose nucleus appear in different forms) in the blood. The lymphocytes, eosinophils (also a leukocyte but one that stains readily with an acid stain, eosin), monocytes and basophils (a type of leukocyte of heavy course granules which stain with basic dyes) decrease in number in the blood stream.

Corticosteroids interfere with a variety of functions, including intra-cellular killing, which is an anti-inflammatory effect. One common mechanism for anti-inflammatory effects is to enhance the production of a specific protein called "lipomodulin," which inhibits "phospholipase A[2]" which in turn is the enzyme necessary for the release of "arachidonic acid" from membrane phospholipids (fatty acid containing phosphorus). Arachidonic acid promotes the "arachidonic cascade" derived prostaglandins effects on cardiovascular, smooth muscle and has other effects. There then follows reduced synthesis of active metabolites (resulting products of the biochemical actions) of arachidonic acid. Arachidonic acid precedes the prostaglandins that result in the inflammatory phenomena. Aspirin and many other non-steroidal anti-inflammatories (NSAIDS) are aimed at inhibiting the production of prostaglandins, which then inhibits the inflammatory symptoms.

The results of all of the phenomena described with such technical medical words is seen mostly in the increased incidence of infection usually controlled by cellular immunity, which means an increase in infections of mycobacterial, fungal, nocardial and cytomegaloviral infections — bacteria, fungus, virus, etc.

Steroids are also used widely in transplantations involving kidney, heart, liver, and bone marrow. In part, subsequent infections that are usually news-media-wise blamed on infections after transplantations is a direct result of use of the corticosteroids as well as other drugs.

Bacterial arthritis is an acute process that occurs in a joint following infection by any one of several microorganisms. Patients who <u>receive</u> intra-articular (in the joint) corticosteroids and those with existing Rheumatoid Arthritis appear to be predisposed to bacterial arthritis. Use of corticosteroids can stimulate and enhance this predisposition.

When corticosteroids result in increased susceptibility to various organisms, the list resembles the agents to which patients with Hodgkin's disease or acquired immune deficiency syndrome (AIDS) are vulnerable. Cryptococcal (fungus infection affecting any organ or tissue) infection is a rare infection overall, but at least half of all patients have some type of immune depression. Steroids can unmask latent Mycobacterium tuberculosis. Nocardial (gram positive bacteria) infections usually involving the lungs or brain occur in patients receiving long-term corticosteroids for a variety of indications (symptoms and signs) including Systemic Lupus Erythmatosus and organ transplantation. *Listeria monocytogenes* causes serious infection in infants who are otherwise healthy and in adults who are immunosuppressed by steroids or lymphreticular (lymph system) malignancy.

There are other negative effects from the use of corticosteroids, but the preceding list should be sufficient to explain why it is necessary to get off of this drug as quickly as possible, and also why the percentage of those helped by our treatment drops drastically when the patient uses some combination of gold, penicillamine, methotrexate and long-term corticosteroids. While I have described the cortisone characteristics, gold, penicillamine and methotrexate, as will be seen, have even worse side-effects.

All of the traditional treatments affect the immunological system in various ways, and the list lengthens as more and more of these damaging medicines are used to suppress symptoms while permitting the disease to rage onward.

All of the forewarnings given were to say this: If you are hooked on cortisone, then start decreasing the dosage, under proper medical supervision. Decreasing the dosage of cortisone can be dangerous if you have reached a stage where daily or weekly shots or oral pills have replaced your body's natural ability to produce cortisol (your body's cortisone). Except for those people who no longer have any ability to produce cortisol for themselves, you MUST get off from any kind of cortisone, whether in the oral form of prednisone or given as injections, or purchased in Mexico under some brand name or through a clinic, or mixed with herbs of various vintage. Again there is another reason, that is, cortisone usage, while damping down symptoms, also permits Arthritis and related diseases to spread. Cortisone also interferes with the effectiveness of our treatment.

If you are on aspirin, or aspirin substitutes called NSAIDS — after the phrase "Non-steroidal Anti-Inflammatory Drugs" — (indomethacin, phenylbutazone, etc.) then you may continue using any of these within safe limits. Their usage will not interfere with the treatments and may not cause your immunological system to weaken. When our treatments are completed successfully you should be pain free, or on minimum dosages of NSAIDS. However persistent reliance on these symptom painkillers can chew up your stomach and create other problems, too.

In our treatment protocol, and on first trial, you should take simultaneously Metronidazole and Allopurinol. Based on a 170 pound weight, you should take 2 grams of Metronidazole either in one dosage, or distributed throughout four equal treatments, per day. You should take this dosage for two days in a row, then skip for five days.

You should repeat this procedure in all for six weeks.

During the first week only, you should take 300 mg of Allopurinol 3 times a day, for 7 days, then quit, taking only the Metronidazole throughout the remaining 5 weeks.

For each 25 pounds you weigh over or under 170 pounds, you should increase or decrease, respectively, your dosage of Metronidazole by 1/4 gram or 250 milligrams.

Five hundred milligram tablets are fine, but if your physician prescribes Metronidazole in 250 mg pills, then you can easily adjust the amount taken by your weight. For example, if you weigh 120 pounds, then you need to reduce the amount taken by 1/2 gram, or two 250 mg tablets, because the difference between 170 pounds and 120 pounds is 50 pounds, which is two 25 pound units less than the treatment formula calls for a 170 pound person. Similarly, therefore, if you weigh 240 pounds, you need to increase the dosage to 2-1/2 grams. A child, therefore, can be administered proper dosage simply by observing the weight and subtracting accordingly. Approximations to the closest 25 pound unit is acceptable.

This technique of dosage by weight is common with prescription writing, because the human body's capability of metabolizing — converting chemicals and food to usable substances, or detoxifying poisons — is often directly correlated to weight.

It happens that all of the 5-nitroimidazoles (Metronidazole, Tinidazole, Clotrimazole, Ornidazole, Nimorazole) are chemically related where, in a five ring nitrogen structure molecule, the first nitrogen position (as defined by organic chemists) is replaced by another set of atoms or molecules. If the resulting molecule is safe for human consumption it also turns out that this is the only nitroimidazole nitrogen substitution that seems to be effective for arthritis without also causing damage. This doesn't mean that others will not be found, nor that some other compounds substituted in the first nitrogen position will not be dangerous. It does mean that so far as we know today, whenever a 5-nitroimidazole compound has the first of five nitrogen atoms replaced, and if the compound is also safe for human use, then it is probably effective for various Rheumatoid Diseases to some degree, and with many people.

Before describing what to expect after taking the above medicines, I will describe the remainder of our protocol, as the effects to be expected are similar in most instances.

If you are one of the rare people allergic to Allopurinol, your doctor may substitute Furazolidone in the following dosage: 100 mg, four times a day for one week only.

Either Allopurinol or Furazolidone may also be taken by themselves as may Metronidazole. However, if you are to benefit by our experiences, it is probably best to take the combination described as first trials.

In the place of Metronidazole, one may take if available any of the other 5-nitroimidazoles, which includes Tinidazole, Clotrimazole, Nimorazole and Ornidazole. They may be taken in combination with Allopurinol or Furazolidone, or by themselves. The dosage is exactly the same as described for Metronidazole, and the time period exactly the same.

Nimorazole and Ornidazole are available in some European countries, and perhaps elsewhere, but not in the United States. Tinidazole is available almost everywhere in the world, and is easily available at any drugstore in Mexico without a prescription under the trade names of Fasigyn or Tinidex. Tindazole and clotrimazole can be ordered with prescription through compounding pharmacies.

Incidentally, the lower cost generic medicines in all of the drugs named is perfectly satisfactory. Diiodohydroxyquinon (known as Iodoquinol) should be taken as 650 mg three times a day, for three weeks.

Potassium Para Amino Benzoate should be taken as 2 grams, 6 times daily for two weeks.

"Copper Ions" are small, resin granules upon which is deposited copper ions by a special process developed by Seldon Nelson, D.O., one of our former referral physicians. Only five one-hundredths of a gram of copper per granule is available. These tiny granules are taken sublingually (beneath the tongue) in various ways: Usually the physician will start the patient with about 20 or 30 granules several times a day, increasing the amount by 10 or 20 per day, until a certain reaction is observed. Since large numbers of these small granules do not exceed the daily minimum requirement for copper, they do not require a prescription. Unfortunately, they cannot be easily obtained, as they were developed by Dr. Seldon Nelson for use with special patients. Dr. Nelson died some years ago and we don't know who is now making the same copper granules.

Rifampin should be taken as 600 mg daily for one month. **Caution on use of this one, as it is a medicine that must be administered under close supervision, and if complications (as to be explained) occur, then the physician should take you off of it immediately.**

If you have nausea with any of these medicines, your physician can prescribe an anti-nausea tablet. I have just described all of the medicines and their dosages in our treatment protocol.

It is best to start with Metronidazole and Allopurinol if possible, but not necessary. It is best to use the various medicines individually or in the combinations already described, but not necessary. Usually most patients respond to the first medicines when used properly in the proper dosages, but there are a significant number that do not. One reason they do not has already been described: their past and possibly present use of gold, penicillamine or methotrexate or long-term cortico-steroids. No one should deny such patients trial with our treatment for those reasons, but they should be made to understand (1) to get off of cortisone if at all possible and safe — and absolutely to get off of gold, penicillamine and methotrexate for 4-months prior to our treatment; and (2) that their response to our treatment may not be as sure, spectacular or swift as those not having been on such drugs; (3) that they may need to use a number of other related and supporting treatments which, by the way, many others may also need in the long run, as will be described.

Prior to taking Metronidazole, the physician should insure that the patient is provided with a good supplement of intestinal microflora, such as *Lactobacilus acidophilus*. Yogurt will not do as it is a bulgaris species. I have other objections to commercial Yogurt, as found in most supermarkets, in that they are often mixed with sugars and promote the growth of a damaging organism called *Candida albicans*, a yeast fungus that can create similar symptoms to Arthritis, and other problems. I also object to the use of pasteurized products labeled as "acidophilus" this or that. If you kill the organisms by pasteurization, then why advertise their presence? (Homogenized milk is another horror story!)

When you look around for a good grade of intestinal microflora supplement use caution. While it does not require a prescription to purchase *Lactibacilus acidophilus* from a health food store, you may be getting a poorly performing species, or, as bad, an organism that has already been weakened by environmental conditions. Any time temperature exceeds about 74 degrees Fahrenheit, the organism may lose viability or die, as when it is transported, left on the floor or in the stockroom of the store temporarily, or inadvertently placed on non-refrigerated shelves. Some non-refrigerated sources are viable, however.

Physicians who administer this beneficial and symbiotic organism usually order from a company that is known to culture a good, viable grade, and it is shipped to you or the physician by overnight air express packed in dry ice, and it is immediately refrigerated, which you will do also on receiving it.

Take about 1/4 teaspoon five or six times daily. Over about three weeks, you should begin to build up proper intestinal microflora so that these organisms will metabolize Metronidazole. Your enzyme system cannot do the job, and that helps to explain why Metronidazole does not always work with Rheumatoid Arthritics in the dosages required. Metronidazole, being also anti-bacterial, may knock out "good guys" microflora on first six-week trials, in which case second-time trials may not be effective, as the "good-guys" microflora is not present in sufficient numbers to metabolize the medicine properly.

Supplementation with viable *Lactobacilus acidophilus* will normalize gut flora and reduce the concentration of gram-negative bacteria, a major source of "endotoxins". Endotoxins are toxins usually confined inside the body of a gram-negative bacterium until it dies, at which time it is released. At the same time Lactibacilus will inhibit overgrowth of *Candida albicans* which has itself been implicated in disruption of immune functions as well as GI inflammation, which could then increase absorption of existing endotoxins.

Such is not true of Clotrimazole and Tinidazole as these similar chemicals can be metabolized by both the human enzyme system and intestinal microflora. It's probably still best to supplement your diet with *Lactibacilus acidophilus* for many reasons, which will be covered later.

As a matter of good practice, after the initial few weeks of build-up of 5 to 6 one-quarter teaspoons per day, it might be well to supplement with the same 1/4 teaspoon about three to four times a day until you are certain that you no longer need the organism or other microflora that your physician may suggest. In any case, it is well to take a dosage with every application of Metronidazole. Your physician may have different dosages in mind, which you should follow.

Incidentally, there is no evidence that Metronidazole when used intravenously has any effect on halting RD, but it does very quickly, and for a period, knock out inflammation that shows itself as swelling and heat. Metronidazole is used intravenously frequently for bacterial infections, especially when the patient has been hospitalized. According to John Baron, D.O., former Rheumatoid Disease Foundation Chairman from Cleveland, Ohio, IVs chiefly affect organs that demand the most blood, such as stomach, duodenum, gall bladder and pancreas. This means that the lower colon and other body portions that receive proportionally less blood will probably not receive sufficient supply of Metronidazole when given through IVs.

The *Physician's Desk Reference* is often mis-interpreted as providing a single standard for administration of drugs, in the belief that only those diseases described therein can be treated by the associated drugs. I want to clarify that this book is simply a collection of drug package inserts placed there by pharmaceutical companies for the benefit of physician, pharmacist and patient in knowing what is being purchased and consumed. These package inserts, with their statements discussing characteristics and possible dangers of taking various medicines, are required by the U.S. Food and Drug Administration.

In addition to scientific findings reported therein, any **possible** danger, whether known to be frequent or not, is contained therein. To gain FDA approval of a particular drug, for the medicinal use the company is promoting, the pharmaceutical company will include many symptoms that seem to occur when taking the drug, including some very rare effects and some symptoms virtually speculative. Whether or not a medicine is traditionally used by physicians for other purposes is seldom mentioned. In particular, if a medicine is being touted by the drug company as, say, an anti-bacterial agent, they have no responsibility to report that it is also used for an anti-protozoal, viral-static, or anti-viral agent.

The *Physician's Desk Reference* is published by Medical Economics Company, Inc., Oradell, N.J. 07649. In it's "Foreword to the Fortieth First Edition" (1987) they state: "The FDA has also announced that the FD & C Act (Federal Drug and Cosmetic Act) 'does not, however, limit the manner in which a physician may use an approved drug. Once a product has been approved for marketing, a physician may prescribe it for uses or in treatment regimens or patient populations that are not included in approved labeling." Thus, the FDA states also that "'accepted medical practice' often includes drug use that is not reflected in approved drug testing."

So, when someone tells you that, say, Metronidazole is an anti-bacterial agent, or that Clotrimazole is mainly an "anti-fungal" agent, and that "everyone knows" that Rheumatoid Arthritis is not caused by bacteria or fungus, just nod and go on your way. Many of the medicines listed above can be shown under laboratory conditions to be combinations of anti-bacterial, anti-viral, viral-static or anti-protozoal or anti-yeast/fungus, under the correct conditions.

In the United States, the most frequently used first-trial medicine for Rheumatoid Disease (RD) is

Metronidazole. It is listed in the *Physician's Desk Reference* as being FDA approved for marketing and human use. It is easily available by prescription and is relatively well known. It's use has resulted in a large number of remissions/cures, including the author's.

However, the medicine of most probable future first-choice is Clotrimazole. While it is available in the United States as an oral tablet for vaginal infections, the mixture of substances in the tablet seem to delay absorption. It is also very costly in that form to obtain the dosage required by our treatment protocol. Under a prescription written by your physician and given to you, Clotrimazole can be obtained through compounding pharmacies. To some extent Clotrimazole is anti-amoebic, anti-viral, viral-static, anti-yeast/fungus, and anti-bacterial. It does not kill all germs, but for certain species, Clotrimazole may be effective in specific dosages under specific conditions.

Clotrimazole also inhibits a substance inside the body known as phospholipase A[2] which is a precursor (forerunner) to production of prostaglandins (from the arachidonic acid cascade) that helps to create inflammatory responses that produce heat (pyrexia), swelling (edema) and pain. Phospholipase is an enzyme derived from a fatty acid containing phosphorus.

Clotrimazole stimulates the body's own production of cortisol. It acts as an "immuno-modulator" changing some of the out-of-kilter characteristics of the immunological system.

It kills *Candida albicans*, the yeast-fungus organism that causes so many symptoms that appear to be Rheumatoid Arthritis, and which also creates other major medical problems which will be explained later.

Clotrimazole is usually easier for the patient to tolerate

than Metronidazole — but patients vary. So, which is the "best" medicine in the whole treatment protocol so far as is known to date? Answer: There is no "best". The medicine that gets you well is best, and that may also vary from person to person.

For now be satisfied that a good honest trial of one (and possibly all) of the given medicines is your "best" opportunity to defeat the crippler than anything else available. Also study and apply the list of treatments for varying causations at the rear of this book.

Chapter V
The Herxheimer Effect

Many traditional medical treatments require a trial and error period, just like ours. the physician evaluates effectiveness of a treatment by observing signs and clinical symptoms, and health progress. With our treatment, both the patient and the physician will know, after starting it, whether or not the treatment will <u>probably</u> be effective.

Usually, when one of the medicines is administered for RD, there will be a set of clinical signs and symptoms called the Jarisch-Herxheimer effect. Observing the Jarisch-Herxheimer effect, hereafter known as "The Herxheimer" is often very important for following the effectiveness of our treatment.

In 1902 two research physicians, Doctors Adolph Jarisch and Karl Herxheimer, studied the treatment of syphilis, using various kinds of relatively dangerous medicines. They learned that whenever they killed the syphilis spirochete the patient displayed a series of symptoms similar to "flu". They later concluded that whenever an organism more complex than a simple bacteria was killed within the human body, one had these same symptoms. Subsequently this phenomenon became named the "Jarisch- Herxheimer" or "Herxheimer" effect.

When treating tuberculosis, the Herxheimer occurs, as it also does in treating Leishmaniasis. When treating Leprosy, the same phenomenon occurs, but it is called "Lucio's" phenomenon". Some other rare, tropical diseases also exhibit the Herxheimer when treated by killing the causative organism.

According to the Jarisch-Herxheimer theory, when an invading organism (more complex than a simple bacteria) acts as an antigen (allergy agent) the body prepares antibodies that tend to fight or neutralize the antigen. This creates products which are the cause of the swelling, heat, and joint damage. One responds to the killing of the organism inside the body by having a serious allergic response inside the body. The products of that allergic response create secondary problems that lead to the additional damage.

If there is a causative organism that creates RD, and if the organism is killed by our medicine, and if a human has been sensitized to the protein products of that organism, then more of the protein products resulting from dead organisms will increase the internal allergic response. It follows, therefore, that the body will have an intensification of the very symptoms that we label as Rheumatoid Arthritis (RA). Rheumatoid Arthritis symptoms are a manifestation of the internal allergy!

Whenever a physician trained in our protocol treats a patient for Rheumatoid Disease, he/she looks very closely to observe if the patient is or is not having a Herxheimer. Usually, within a matter of a day or so the Herxheimer will occur if the treatment is to be successful. Such generality cannot be a golden rule, because there are a number of former arthritics who have had to take the medicine as long as six or seven weeks prior to observing a Herxheimer, and some few have Herxheimer's that do not seem to terminate.

There are some, like I was, who are so sick at the time of treatment that neither the doctor nor patient are able to discriminate between the on-going disease and the Herxheimer. That is rare, however, and the normal case that is to respond will show the Herxheimer within a matter of days of treatment. A very few patients will get better without experiencing anything but a very light Herxheimer — which they might not notice — but this is not the norm.

As reported by Gus J. Prosch, M.D. of Birmingham, AL, the Herxheimer signs and symptoms are:

a. General and usual: Sweating and especially night sweats, diarrhea, nausea, vomiting, headache, fever, general malaise, flushing of skin, anorexia, aching bones and "flu" symptoms resembling a serum reaction.

b. The inflamed and affected tissues become more inflamed and tissues previously unknown to be involved become inflamed.

c. If the heart, pericardium or cardiac tissues are infected, patients may develop some paroxysmal auricular tachycardia, premature ventricular contractions or ectopic beats.

d. If the urinary bladder tissues are infected the patient may develop signs of full-blown cystitis.

e. If the brain or meninges are infected the patient may develop severe (temporary) depression, lethargy, generalized weakness, temporary memory loss, irritability along with headaches.

f. If the mouth tissues are infected, a bitter and/or

38

metallic taste may be noted along with mild shedding or peeling of the mucosal tissues. This has also been noted in the rectal tissues. However, <u>it should be noted that Metronidazole and Tinidazole also produce a metallic taste without the Herxheimer effect</u> being present.

g. When the periosteal tissues and skeletal muscle tissues are involved, fairly severe bone pain usually accompanied by severe muscle pains and spasms may be observed, usually at night.

h. When the lungs and bronchial tissues are infected the patients may develop bronchitis symptoms and occasionally pneumonitis (resembling viral) has been observed.

From the above, Dr. Prosch states, one can easily see that most all of the previously observed side effects of the recommended medicines may also be simply manifestations of the Herxheimer reaction. Therefore a clinician that is not totally knowledgeable concerning these possible signs and symptoms could easily mistake the Herxheimer reaction for possible side effects of the medicine. Should this information not be taken into consideration, a misleading and false evaluation of any adverse experiences by various patients caused by the medicine will be inevitable. The medicine could be labeled more dangerous than it actually may be, and the aggravated symptoms could get misconstrued as an intensification of the disease being treated. The information and the above facts **must be considered** in evaluating the medicine's effectiveness and side effects, when treating patients.

While the medicines may have a toxicity of their own — and in large dosages they surely do have — the symptoms listed in the *Physician's Desk Reference* are probably in many instances a report on the Herxheimer reaction rather than actual drug toxicity. The proof is that when a patient takes the medicine, and passes through the Herxheimer, the same drug dosage no longer produces the symptoms described on the package insert.

Professor Roger Wyburn-Mason's hypothesis that there exists a causative organism for Rheumatoid Disease which is more complex than a simple bacteria bears fruit. Once the Herxheimer is achieved, and the body cleans out the dead protein products (if that is what they are) and toxins, the individual gets well; i.e., the symptoms of swelling (edema), heat (pyrexia) and increasing number of joint pains disappear, along with lethargy and depression.

From personal experience, and even though I knew full well better, during a course of a particular medicine, I have condemned and blamed the medicine as being the "cause" of my agony, the Herxheimer. Afterwards, on cleaning out the debris within my body, I have felt wonderful, and the medicine in the same dosage is now seen as obviously not the cause of the Herxheimer. "Cleaning out the debris" means giving the body an opportunity to metabolize and/or eliminate toxins and other allergenic products.

"Double-blind" studies were mentioned in the foregoing. While it is not entirely necessary in every scientific study, it is usually the standard accepted by the scientific medical community. A practicing physician could have treated 16,000 patients with great effectiveness, as did Jack Blount, Jr., M.D. prior to his retirement. Sixteen thousand, 20,000, . . . 100,000 patients are meaningless to the scientific medical community, unless those studies have been cast in the framework of double-blind studies, and subsequently accepted for publication in an accepted "peer-group", "refereed" medical journal. "Refereed" means that "peer" scientific physicians have an opportunity to search for scientific flaws in the article prior to being accepted for publication. Even then the publisher of a particular medical journal may not, for reasons of bias or space or unknown reasons, reject the article for publication.

You can understand, then, that there is a great deal of political jockeying for space in such "peer group" journals, as publication therein can make reputations and lead to better position and pay. There will be a tendency to build up respectability via the "buddy-buddy" system, as well as by "Authority," through "co-authoring" one another's articles. A big name on an article, along with the investigator's, assures publication and often acceptance by the scientific community. The more a scientist gets published, the easier it is for the scientist to get published.

An ordinary practitioner of medicine has about as much chance of getting published in such "peer" group journals as the proverbial snowball surviving a day in hades, especially so when their chief dedication is toward helping patients, not in becoming an Authority.

What follows introduces patient treatment studies completed in a clinical setting by three different physicians in three different locations, with three different practices. Each physician making his own study wanted to satisfy himself that they were helping folks, and so, for their own purposes, they accumulated statistics in a setting that is not accepted as "proof" by authoritarian standards or "accepted" "peer-group" standards.

Dr. Jack M. Blount's clinical work is not included for other reasons told in detail in *Rheumatoid Diseases Cured at Last!*

Briefly, Dr. Blount had had crippling Rheumatoid Disease since childhood. When he discovered Roger Wyburn- Mason's work, he was already bed-ridden, unable to walk, alcoholic, on drugs to kill the eternal pain and prepared to die. Trials of Metronidazole made him well. He called in a dozen elderly former patients giving them the opportunity to try the drug. Most of those who stayed with the treatment also got well. He reopened his practice and treated with great effectiveness another group of RD patients in excess of 16,000, including myself. As a former RD victim Dr. Blount was more familiar with the disease and its progress than most physicians, and it was quite obvious to him that the treatment was working on the vast majority of his patients.

William Renforth, M.D. of Connersville, IN reported his studies in 1977. They are also not included, but can be obtained from this Foundation. Go online and see Historical Documents in Search for the Cure for Rheumatoid Disease.

Gus J. Prosch, Jr. (deceased) had a successful medical trial on his back problem that traditional practices stated would require an operation. Dr. Blount had suggested he try Metronidazole and Allopurinol first, as Dr. Prosch could always have the operation if the medicine did not help. The treatment was successful in ridding Dr. Prosch of his back pain for the first time in 7 years. On behalf of his patients, Dr. Prosch felt an obligation to study his case histories and to compile their statistics.

Another of our referral physicians, Robert Bingham, M.D., (deceased) on the other hand, had specialized as an orthopaedic surgeon and general practitioner with polio victims and later arthritic victims, the latter for more than 30 years. He therefore knew success and non-success quite well. Through his long years of experience he further had an ability to separate out various kinds of arthritic characteristics (signs and symptoms) and could, therefore, pre-select patients who would most likely respond to Rheumatoid Disease protocols.

Dr. Paul K. Pybus, (deceased) our Chief Medical Advisor, worked under the supervision of Roger Wyburn-Mason, M.D. (deceased) in his youth, and had learned to respect the physician's brilliance and originality in medicine. Pybus investigated Wyburn-Mason's claims, tried the treatments, and was convinced by his patient results. Dr. Pybus often publishes his observations as "Letters" in the *South African Medical Journal* or the English published *Lancet*.

Statistics compiled by Prosch, Bingham and Pybus follow:

PARTIAL REPORT OF
SUMMARY OF TREATING PATIENTS WITH MEDICATION
Gus J. Prosch, Jr., M.D.

Effect	Metronidazole	%	Furoxone	%	Rimactane	%
None	7	3.5	23	39.0	16	5.0
Mild	9	4.5	7	11.9	5	16.0
Moderate			29	14.5	5	8.5
	3	9.0				
Good	56	28.0	14	23.7	5	16.0
Very Good			99	49.5	1 0	1 6 . 9
	3	9.0				
Total	**200**	**100**	**59**	**100**	**32**	**55**

COMPARATIVE RESULTS OF TREATMENT WITH OTHER DRUGS

Robert Bingham, M.D.

Treatment	Patients Treated	Improved or Remissions	Percent Change
Controls	22	7	31
Conventional Care	30	8	27
Copper Sulfate	12	8	66
Bile Salts	12	9	75
Clotrimazole	9	7	78
Diiodohydroxyquinon	204	189	93
Chloroquine	12	6	50
Metronidazole	221	181	82*

*Recent cases have done better on increased dosages.

CLINICAL RESULTS IN 156 PATIENTS

Dr. Paul K. Pybus

Clinical Results	Number	Percent
Poor (no change)	11	7
Fair (slightly improved)	35	22
Good (one joint still troublesome)	60	38
Excellent (symptomless)	50	32

Nearly four years (1992) have passed since these studies were made. Subsequent follow-up data passed to me orally from those physicians who tally their clinical results indicate a <u>consistent</u> 80% success rate in patient populations, the one exception being the 50% sub-group success rate noted for those that have already been abused by gold, penicillamine, methotrexate and long-term cortico-steroids.

Earlier I reported on the "placebo" effect in the treating of arthritics, and that it was 30%. This means that any scientific statistical study must account for about 30% of the patients responding well — or at least appearing to — for reasons to do with mood, natural variations between humans, "belief" or "faith" or reasons just unknown. No matter what a physician does the patient will show "improvement" at least temporarily.

Look closely at the statistics offered. Study them. There can be no explanation for the great differences between an anticipated placebo effect of 30% and the <u>consistent</u> 80% success rate, or better displayed by different physicians in far different clinical settings with much different backgrounds and experiences! — other than to conclude the extremely high probability that the treatment protocol is 165% or greater better than traditional treatments, and safer than traditional Rheumatology practices which, remember, do not claim to cure or permanently improve anyone, but do claim to get about 30% "improvement," at least temporarily. Note that the 30% placebo effect is exactly the same figure as the 30% temporary "improvement" effect achieved in traditional practices. For the source of the 30% figure, read *Clinics in Rheumatic Diseases*, December 1983, published by W.B. Saunders, a peer-group accepted publication informing practicing rheumatologists of the state-of-art of their treatment protocols as scientifically evaluated.

There are some patients, it should be mentioned in passing, who will get well permanently no matter what is done. Medical science does not explain this, other than to label it as a "spontaneous remission" which is a scientific name substituted for the term "faith cure" used by various religious groups.

We are quite happy for wellness in former victims, no matter how labeled or to whom they attribute their great relief.

Chapter VI
How Dangerous Are the Recommended Medicines?

Physicians have observed that the more severe the Herxheimer, the more probability, and degree, of wellness.

We do not recommend use of cortisone to cover up these temporary symptoms, but sometimes it is necessary to do so because of the severity of the Herxheimer reaction, or because the reaction is so severe as to interfere with the patient's ability to work.

We try to get the patient to use our portion of the treatment protocol entitled "Intraneural Injections", rather than oral or injected "systemic" cortisone. The intra-neurals do not act systemically, and they get at the pain's source immediately, also halting the pain at once.

We do not encourage the continued use of cortisone in any form. It only sustains the disease of Rheumatoid Arthritis, and it also weakens the immunological system in other ways, and further permits the spread of Candidiasis that results from a common yeast/fungus organism, with other consequences, as will be discussed later.

In the dosages specified by our treatment protocol,

physicians have not seen any serious side effects of the medicines. I am at the hub of both Foundation research findings and patient complaints as well as their successes. I've talked to several patients who have gone out on their own, without physician sanction and supervision, and have overdosed themselves, such is their drive to change their terrible pain.

Their body has responded in this mis-treatment by creating peripheral neuropathy and paresthesia. The extremities burn, nerves convey a tingling sensation and other unusual feelings. Some damage has been done to the nerves and it may take as long as seven years for damaged nerve cells to repair, and for one to lose these uncomfortable, often painful sensations.

When this phenomena begins in a patient, it is not the Herxheimer, and the physician knows to take the patient off from the dosage or the medicine immediately, in which case there is no permanent damage, and the sensations will restore immediately.

The reason that Rimactane is a "last resort" medicine is because overdose, for a sensitive person, can produce these sensations quite apart from a most severe Herxheimer, and the physician must supervise closely to insure that the patient is not so affected. There is no danger if taken under close medical supervision.

Any medicine, even the most innocuous, can be misused. Our recommended medicines have now been prescribed and taken by tens of thousands without undue affects, other than the Herxheimer. Our recommended medicines are certainly far, far safer than poisons traditionally used, involving gold, penicillamine, methotrexate and cortico-steroids.

For example, I quote from the *Physician's Desk*

Reference on the use of Methotrexate:

WARNING

METHOTREXATE MUST BE USED ONLY BY PHYSICIANS EXPERIENCED IN ANTIMETABOLITE CHEMOTHERAPY.

BECAUSE OF THE POSSIBILITY OF FATAL OR SEVERE TOXICITY REACTIONS, THE PATIENT SHOULD BE FULLY INFORMED BY THE PHYSICIAN OF THE RISKS INVOLVED AND SHOULD BE UNDER HIS CONSTANT SUPERVISION. IN THE TREATMENT OF PSORIASIS, METHOTREXATE SHOULD BE RESTRICTED TO SEVERE, RECALCITRANT, DISABLING PSORIASIS WHICH IS NOT ADEQUATELY RESPONSIVE TO OTHER FORMS OF THERAPY, BUT ONLY WHEN THE DIAGNOSIS HAS BEEN ESTABLISHED AS BY BIOPSY AND OR AFTER DERMATOLOGIC CONSULTATION.

1. Methotrexate may produce marked depression of bone marrow, anemia, leukopenia, thrombocytopenia and bleeding.

2. Methotrexate may be hepatotoxic, particularly at high dosage or with prolonged therapy. Liver atrophy, necrosis, cirrhosis, fatty changes, and periportal fibrosis have been reported. Since changes may occur without previous signs of gastrointestinal or hematologic toxicity, it is imperative that hepatic function be determined prior to initiation of treatment and monitored regularly throughout therapy. Special caution is indicated in the presence of pre-existing liver damage or impaired hepatic function. Concomitant use of other drugs with hepatotoxic potential (including alcohol) should be avoided.

3. Methotrexate has caused fetal death and/or congenital anomalies. Therefore, it is not recommended in women of childbearing potential unless there is appropriate medical evidence that the benefits can be expected to outweigh the considered risks. Pregnant psoriatic patients should not receive Methotrexate.

4. Impaired renal function is usually contraindication.

5. Diarrhea and ulcerative stomatis are frequent toxic effects and require interruption of therapy; otherwise hemorrhagic enteritis and death from intestinal perforation may occur.

METHOTREXATE HAS BEEN ADMINISTERED IN VERY HIGH DOSAGE FOLLOWED BY LEUCOVORIN RESCUE IN EXPERIMENTAL TREATMENT OF CERTAIN NEOPLASTIC DISEASES. THIS PROCEDUR IS INVESTIGATIONAL AND HAZARDOUS.

If you have followed the blighted history of attempts to conquer Cancer, then you know that billions have been spent for more than two generations following the "cut, slash and burn" (surgery, chemotherapy, radiation medical procedures), to little effect. Now, after killing tens of thousands through blindness and prejudice, and with surgery, chemotherapy and radiation, those in financial power are at last admitting that nutritional components and other preventive measures are effective cancer prevention measures, as has long been claimed by various alternative medical practitioners.

Proper diet for arthritics is also essential, as we will later discuss.

Similar blindness and prejudice, based on Authoritarian claims and status, cause psychiatrists to cut out portions of the brain or fry and to scramble the brain with electric shock and other forms of destructive therapy, because they lacked any true knowledge of mind/brain processes.

Heart by-pass surgery suffers for the most part from the same blindness and prejudices, even after prominent medical leaders, such as Debakey, have shown that statistics generally do not support heart by-pass surgery. Others have demonstrated that Chelation Therapy — more on this later — solves the problem of peripheral circulation and 80% of carotid artery problems, and similar circulatory problems with a high frequency, and also reverses osteoporosis. Chelation therapy is extremely easy to use, safe and low cost when compared to generally ineffective by-pass surgery.

Now, after years of mis-using arthritics through gold, penicillamine and long-term cortico-steroids, the "in-thing" to do is to treat us Arthritics with Methotrexate!?

A Rheumatoid Disease patient would have to have a deeply embedded death wish to agree to submit to this form of treatment!!

Sometimes a patient who has received our treatment continues to have a Herxheimer reaction throughout the sixth week of treatment. According to our treatment protocol, the physician should continue the treatment for further weeks, sometimes throughout another six week term, with either the Furazolidone or Allopurinol continued for the specified time periods for each, as reported earlier, and along with one of the nitroimidazoles.

With a patient who has received our treatment and does not respond throughout the six week treatment, we recommend rotation to another medicine on our list, in search by trial and error of a medicine that will create the desired Herxheimer and improvement.

I know one person who tried every single medicine except one, and he had avoided that one because last time he had had it prescribed for a totally different medical purpose he'd had an "allergic" reaction to it, breaking out in a severe rash.

Normally medicines that produce an allergic rash are to be avoided, but part of the Herxheimer reaction FOR THIS PARTICULAR PERSON was to have a skin rash. When his physician learned about the "allergic" reaction to the medicine, the patient was immediately placed on it. The patient got sicker than he'd been in years with RD. He vomited, broke out with a terrible skin rash, could not work, developed terrible joint pains, and so on. Within weeks he was at last well.

Such a severe reaction is really "good news" as severity of reaction is directly proportional to degree of wellness.

Unfortunately I cannot recommend that you take any medicine that creates an allergy condition, because it might be just that — an allergy. And, without close medical supervision, you could endanger yourself.

A point is proved. Not all formerly observed reactions to a medicine are necessarily toxicities or allergies to the medicine, but may very well be the Herxheimer reaction where, if permitted to continue would lead to wellness.

A baby can be born dead from Rheumatoid Disease. A child can be so affected by RD that it may never learn to walk, especially when treated by traditional methods. Such a child is in habitual pain and there lives cannot be anything but pure, unadulterated agony.

Young people in their teens can develop the disease, and so can middle-aged and aged.

We have learned that the earlier our treatment is tried,

after finding that you have the disease, the more probability of success in halting its progress. This is true for age, too, in that the earlier in life one comes to our treatment, usually the more quickly is the disease halted, and the more quickly that damage is repaired.

In the case of older people, when they come to us early without considerable damage to their various bodily systems, opportunity exists for stopping the disease progress. The longer they wait, or the more ineffective treatments they take — which also contributes to the damage done during the waiting period — the more damage to the bodily repair systems, and less likelihood of being able to make a significant change.

When a young person or child develops the disease, parents will naturally sacrifice to help that child on the road to health by finding "the very best physician or clinic possible". The very best physician or clinic will give traditional "peer-group-accepted" treatments, which means: first aspirin, then non-steroidal anti-inflammatories (NSAIDS), then cortisone, then gold, penicillamine, and finally methotrexate — all in order as the disease continues onward.

In a vote not long ago rheumatologists voted to reverse this insane protocol by starting arthritics with the most damaging drug first, methotrexate!

By the time the parents get wise to the fact that their child will not recover under such treatments, and in fact is getting worse each week, and only after having spent thousands of dollars do these otherwise — understandably — well-meaning parents begin looking for alternative therapies to produce a kind of miracle.

It is only then that their minds and heart are willing to listen and to try advice by the "non-authority", the practitioners of alternative medicines.

We know that if a younger person has just developed the disease, and if their body is otherwise healthy, they will respond to our treatment with a success rate far higher than our average 80%

We also know that as a person gets older, success figures decline, because — as has been stated — other necessary bodily functions for wellness also decline.

Eighty-six percent of Prosch's patients were 50 years and older — and still the statistics reflected an average of 80% improvement and/or cure.

There are other treatments that will assist this protocol to work on you more effectively, and those will be taken up next. Also additional primary causations and treatments will be taken up at the rear of this book.

I wish that I could say that everyone will be cured, and that we never fail. No field of medicine can make such a claim. I can guarantee this: the sooner you try our treatment after learning that you've developed Rheumatoid Arthritis — no matter your age — the higher probability of getting you totally well!

I have received many letters from elderly in nursing homes — eighties or nineties — who are depressed from the fact that their physician — which they seldom see — refuses to give them anything at all because of their age, and they lay in dismal pain waiting to die. Callousness is one thing, denying our treatment another. If the physical body can tolerate any of our medicines, it ought to be tried at any age, and if not, surely there are better answers than permitting an aged one to lay endlessly in pain —!

Chapter VII
Intraneural Injections — Part of Foundation

Protocol

An extremely important addition and adjunct to our treatment protocol is the use of intraneural injections as developed by Pybus/Wyburn-Mason/Prosch. Arthritics get better faster when this treatment is used, as there is immediate relief of pain and discomfort and often relief of crippling effects. Unfortunately not all of our referral physicians are versed in this treatment. A physician needs a good knowledge of anatomy to apply the treatment, and many are reluctant to perform the tasks without having had direct supervision from a knowledgeable physician.

Professor Roger Wyburn-Mason was initially a specialist in nerve diseases, and he demonstrated for Dr. Pybus, who was then his "House Physician," (like an intern) that one could use alcohol and deaden key nerve locations, thus eliminating the pain of certain arthritic symptoms at once. Unfortunately the alcohol itself was exceedingly painful, and there was no substance fifty years ago that was known by the two that could do the same job effectively.

Over thirty years were to pass before Pybus serendipitously discovered a means of implementing Wyburn-Mason's findings.

According to Pybus' theory, certain key nerve locations, called "neuromata" serve as trigger points for creating a kind of nerve signal "confusion" to portions of the anatomy. When nerves have damage or lesions at these locations, one set of impulses travels directly to the spinal cord where a reflex arc, not unlike that which draws your hand away from a hot surface when touched, sends signals back to the joints served by those nerves, causing muscles at the joint to contract and create spasms. The spasms cause the joint to compress together and cause damage to the underlying cartilage. The cartilage requires a compression and expansion action — not unlike a sponge — to supply it with nourishment from two sources: diffusion from vessels through bone marrow, and circulation of synovial fluid at the surface of the cartilage. When the cartilage is squeezed (by motion of the joint), synovial fluid moves out, taking away waste products. When it is expanded, fluids move in, supplying nourishment. A healthy joint must expand and contract, whereas an unhealthy joint will result when the joint is "frozen" by continuous traction or stiffness caused by damaged muscles or inflamed nerves. When the joint compresses causing damage to the underlying cartilage it is known as Osteoarthrosis. At the time a barrage of signals also travels to brain and back (peripherally) creating inflammation, and this is known as Osteoarthritis.

So long as there is a disturbance in the nerves as cited, this condition persists. It can, therefore, be seen as a similar condition insofar as pain and cartilage deterioration occur in both Rheumatoid Disease and Osteoarthritis, although the causes may not be the same.

Dr. Prosch and Dr. Blount have found that a very small percentage of Osteoarthritis is a secondary condition stemming from a primary condition of Rheumatoid Disease and Dr. Prosch will therefore as a precautionary measure treat both Osteoarthritis and Rheumatoid Arthritis with the Rheumatoid Disease oral medication while also treating with intraneural injections, which relieves the pain in both instances.

The nerves that bear the damage, whether biochemical or mechanical (as in sports injuries), usually are the so-called C-fibres or unmyelinated fibres. "Unmyelinated" means that the nerves do not have an insulated sheath. They are usually found near the skin's surface. The A-fibres or myelinated nerves do have an insulation and are buried more deeply, as a rule, but they sometimes run together with the C-fibres.

The C-fibres are damaged more easily. Throughout the body these inflamed points may be found by "palpating" which means to press either a thumb or eraser on a pencil to find tender spots.

Most of the recommended intraneural locations correspond exactly with ancient acupuncture points, but not all of them. Dr. Pybus also has shown the theoretical relationship between the use of acupuncture and the development of intraneurals, each having their place in treatment to relieve pain.

For details on the Foundation's treatment and theory behind it, we recommend requesting the book

Intraneural Injections for Rheumatoid Arthritis and The Control of Pain in Arthritis of the Knee (ISBN: 0-931150-14-0) by Paul Notrik (Dr. Pybus's pseudonym to keep him out of supposed medical ethic problems, as defined in South Africa. This book is available on Kindle or Nook and soon to be available as a book through Createspace.)

A number of physicians have interpreted Pybus's intraneurals as being simply nerve blocks, sclerotherapy, or neural therapy. It is none of these. Each of these valid treatment forms has their own place in medical practice.

Continuing with description of the Wyburn-Mason/Pybus/Prosch treatment, the physician palpates, i.e., presses with thumb or eraser, and finds points along the nerve pathway that are exceedingly sensitive compared to other locations along the nerve. He marks these positions on the skin. Then he desensitizes the skin at each mark. Finally he injects a mixture of pain killer such as procaine along with Aristospan, a "depot" form of cortisone that does not act systemically. The "depot" form stays in the location required to heal cellular lesions at that position.

When the hyperdermic needle is inserted at one of the marked positions, he may have to probe lightly with the point until the inflamed nerve is located. When it is found, you will feel a very sharp pain sensation and you'll be able immediately to tell the physician "That's it!'

The physician then injects the mixture. In about 1-1/2 hours the pain-killing effect of the procaine, lidocaine or zyolcaine wears off. That spot may be moderately painful for about two days, but the pain of the arthritis at the joint will disappear virtually at once. People have thrown away their crutches or wheelchairs at this point, and walked out of the physician's office!

About the third day the moderate pain of the injection wears off. If a very small needle like those used by dentists is used, the pain and bruise resulting from the injection will be minimal, and will be barely perceptible.

If the treatment is wholly effective there will be complete pain relief for an indefinite period. Pybus' statistics follow:

Survey of Intraneural Therapy Cases in Files A-G
Dr. Paul K. Pybus

Type of Joint (Months)	Numbers of Numbers	Months of Failures	Average Relief of joint pain Relief
Hips	37	3	385	10.4
Knees		124	7	

1421	11.4					
Ankles	44	5	491		11.1	
Shoulders	44		1		716	16.3
Elbows		19		0	339	7.3
Hands	56	7	549		9.6	
Sciatica		20		2	283	14.2
Totals	**393**	**25**	**4740**		**11.3**	

Only those patients who have been regularly followed up are included. There are many other patients whose results we do not have, as the patients have been lost to follow-up.

In my personal experience, these treatments were a blessing for three years. I found that each time that I had them (about 6-9 months apart) there were less sensitive locations to treat, and those that were treated lasted longer. I was fortunate in that Dr. Gus Prosch, Jr. of Birmingham, AL was willing to treat me as required, and everyone is fortunate in that he was also willing to teach other physicians.

Dr. Paul Pybus had since learned that one should not give up on reducing the pain (and subsequent crippling) by means of these treatments until at least three times have been tried to no good effect.

Some key locations will have their pain resolved immediately, depending upon their nature. Some locations will require longer. Some may never become resolved because they represent damage or on-going processes for which intraneurals behave no better and last no longer than ordinary nerve blocks.

Dr. Gus Prosch, and other physicians who use this

treatment with our oral medications have learned that patients respond better and often faster to our oral medication than if they had not had the intraneurals.

I must recommend that you either educate your family doctor to these good findings, or find a physician who will give them and knows how to do them satisfactorily.

The average length of time that the pain has been relieved, from the population group studied, is one year. This figure has included both Osteoarthritis and Rheumatoid Arthritis.

From personal experience, it is clear that unless the causation has been removed, the pain will recur at the time the Aristospan wears off, or in about 3 weeks. But — as I've stated — every time I had these injections (usually, and gratefully, by Dr. Prosch) they lasted longer and there were less key locations to do. I remember one trip to Dr. Prosch where I could hardly walk on one knee. I went dancing that night after his treatment, and I danced rather vigorously. That knee has not bothered me for many years — but other points, such as the shoulder and hip, required intraneurals about every six months.

The length of time that a treatment will be effective depends on many factors: state of health generally, nature of nutritional intake, whether or not suffering from recurring arthritis, and so on.

Independent confirmation of Dr. Paul K. Pybus' intraneural injection procedures has been received from Isaac Henry John Bourne, M.D. of the United Kingdom. Dr. Bourne had for a number of years used techniques virtually identical to Pybus, and his latest write-up can be found in the Handbook of Chronic Pain Management Burrows, Elton, Stanley, Eds., Elsevier Science Publishers Biomedical Division, under the title of "The General

Practitioner and Management of Chronic Pain" (E.R. Squibb and Sons Limited, Squibb House, 141/;149 Staines Road, Hounslow, TW3 3JA, England).

The purpose of the Aristospan is to heal cell lesions in the key neuromata from which stems signals that create the tension and inflammation. If the source of those cell lesions is not solved, the pain and lesions will return. Again, as stated, Pybus has found that one should try the injections at a site three tries before giving up on them.

It should be again emphasized that using these injections by themselves, in the absence of other necessary treatments, including ours for Rheumatoid Disease, is not going to stop the progress of Rheumatoid Disease.

I no longer have the severe shoulder and hip pain, but rather have problems in the spine, one shoulder (at a different location) and neck pain that I'm trying to solve through another approach, which will be covered later. Since the intraneurals are not successful at these new locations, the pain is probably due to calcium spurs irritating nerves that stem from the spine, or torn ligatures, tendons or muscle connections to bone.

After halting the progress of Rheumatoid Disease in myself, I discovered that one joint on one little finger would not quit its inflammation and subsequent damage leading to deformity. Intra-neurals also would not stop it.

I later learned that three treatments of "EDTA Chelation Therapy" stopped it completely for the first time in over two years of trying many different kinds of treatment. More on Chelation later.

What I have said about Rheumatoid Disease also applies to the pain of Osteoarthritis, except that the underlying causes may be different. In which case, the pains may or may not return after injections, depending upon whether or not the true underlying causes for the nerve lesions are uncovered for each condition.

It is very important to understand that we do not recommend the use of cortisone ordinarily, and we especially do not recommend its use directly into joints, as the practice gives but symptomatic relief and also damages the joints.

We do not recommend nerve blocks, as the practice does not give more than a handful of days pain- free, and does not address the source of joint disturbance.

You must know clearly that joint pains for the most part derive from these damaged nerves, not from something inherently wrong with the joint!

Chapter VIII
Candidiasis

A treatment that virtually all arthritics should consider as part of their overall "get well" program, and to be used simultaneously with The Rheumatoid Disease Foundation protocol, is that against Candidiasis. Candidiasis, a yeast/fungus organism that seems to be everywhere, was first defined as a set of manifesting symptoms or syndrome by Dr. Orion Truss, M.D. of Birmingham, Al.

Subsequent investigations by many physicians seems to have verified Truss's findings, and slowly but surely it is being accepted by the ultra-conservative medical establishment as a properly defined and diagnosed disease.

Candida albicans invades various parts of bodily tissues, resulting in localized infections. Common sites of infection are the mouth as in infant Thrush, gastrointestinal tract, vagina, urinary tract, prostate gland

and skin and fingernails and toenails.

Under normal conditions your body is able to resist this invasion, as it does other germs. However, whenever various substances weaken the immunological system, the yeast/fungus organism begins to spread, and in the spreading creates virtual havoc throughout the body parts and systems.

The yeast/fungus invasion may cripple the immune system so that it can no longer repel invaders. It can create allergies to chemicals and foods. It is believed that it invades the intestinal wall where toxins from microorganisms and protein molecules from your food enter the blood stream, being there recognized by antibodies as a foreign antigen. Because proteins are derived from common DNA (gene molecule) structure, each time a new protein enters directly into the bloodstream, it, too, can become recognized as a foreign invader, and thus a "cross-reactivity" occurs, causing one to have increasingly more food allergies.

Yeast, remember, feeds on sugars and carbohydrates that easily convert to sugars. In turn, yeasts produce a series of chemical products as waste among which are acetaldehyde and ethanol. Ethanol is alcohol, and there are cases of people on record who have never drunk a drop of alcohol yet are daily inebriated. Acetaldehyde is produced as the alcohol breaks down and is about six times more toxic to brain tissue than ethanol. These two chemicals are probably responsible for the following effects, according to Dr. Orion Truss:

1. Cell membrane defects, damage to red and white blood cells and other problems.

2. Enzyme destruction. Enzymes are the key to breaking down foods in the body so that they can be

utilized as nourishment.

3. Abnormal hormone response. Hormones regulate your bodily functions. Some of the symptoms caused by *Candida albicans* are these:

1. Allergic reactions.

2. Gastrointestinal problems: bloating and gas, diarrhea, abdominal pain, gastritis, gastric ulcers, constipation, and many others.

3. Respiratory system: sore throat, sore mouth, contribution to sinus infections, bronchial infections and pneumonia.

4. Cardiovascular system. palpitations, rapid pulse rate, pounding heart.

5. Genitourinary system: vaginitis, frequent urination, lack of bladder control, itchy rashes, etc.

6. Musculoskeletal system: muscle weakness, leg pains, muscle stiffness, slow coordination, and so on.

7. Central Nervous system: Headaches, poor brain function, poor short-term memory, fuzzy thinking and so on.

8. Fatigue is extremely common as impaired metabolism doesn't enable the body to get enough fuel and impaired enzyme functioning inhibits energy production.

9. Weight gain is common.

As can be observed by reviewing the above characteristic symptoms (which are not complete) many similar symptoms may "present" with Rheumatoid Disease. It is often difficult to discriminate between one cause and another as different diseases operate on the same tissues, the same organs, producing similar symptoms, in similar ways.

I recommend that you read the book *The Yeast*

Syndrome, John Parks Trowbridge, M.D. and Morton Walker, D.P.M.and other books on candidiasis found in many publication lists, especially those of William Crook, M.D.

Rheumatoid Disease spreads with a weakening of the immunological system. *Candida albicans* spreads with a weakening of the immunological system.

Rheumatoid Disease as well as Candidiasis seems to lead to food allergies and other kinds of allergies over time.

Both diseases produce similar symptoms in many bodily tissues. Both diseases are systemic in nature.

A Candidiasis victim does not necessarily have Rheumatoid Disease, but a Rheumatoid Disease victim almost certainly suffers from Candidiasis.

Candidiasis spreads with the use of almost any kind of surgery where antibiotics were used, or if you've been given antibiotics orally for any purpose, you probably suffer from some degree of Candidiasis. Why? Because the antibiotics kill off the "good-guys" bacteria required in your intestinal tract for good nutrition, the yeast/fungus spreads, taking the "good-guys'" place, and sending rootlets into the intestinal mucosa, and helping to age your total system. Candidiasis also takes hold and spreads under long term stress, and through use of hormonal pills, such as those used for birth control.

Candidiasis is usually controlled through a combination of diet control and medicines some of which are prescription and some non-prescription. Usually the physician who suspects Candidiasis also attempts to strengthen the immunological system by one means or another.

It is important to replace the yeast in the intestinal

tract with Lactobacili as well. Remember my earlier recommendation to use *Lactobacilus acidophilus* when taking medicines we recommend for Rheumatoid Disease? We stated that this supplemental organism helped to metabolize certain medicines, like Metronidazole. Here is another reason to take it. *Lactobacilus acidophilus* helps digest food and especially milk sugar. Some varieties also synthesize vitamin B and some reduce serum cholesterol levels.

While increasingly mounting evidence is being accumulated by establishment medical practitioners that Candidiasis is a real syndrome, much controversy still exists. Allergists, immunologists, and gynecologists see this syndrome as a fictional one, probably because the manifestations are seen too often, the treatments too frequent, the traditional testing for its presence and effect too inadequate, and because almost everyone suddenly has become an expert in its presence or absence.

Most determination for the presence of Candidiasis takes place by means of a questionnaire which the patient fills out and is then evaluated by either a physician or a medical technician. If a score of a certain amount is reached, one is at risk for having the syndrome, otherwise probably not.

There are accredited laboratories that perform accurate, objective testing for the presence of the organism. Such tests may be done in two stages, the first called the Micro-ELISA technique that detects circulating levels of Candida antigens, Candida antibodies IgG, IgA and IgM, and immune complexes. In the second stage of the test, the patient's lymphocytes (white cells) are challenged with Candida to evaluate inhibition of lymphocyte multiplication by budding (blastogenesis).

According to one medical doctor, Candidiasis was adequately treated in those patients who tested positive by the above test within three months by use of Ketoconazole, without any diet being required. He felt that it was "ludicrous to assume that one can 'starve Candida out' by avoidance of sugar, yeast and moldy foods". (Ketoconazole is not one of our recommended 5-nitroimidazoles used for Rheumatoid Disease treatment, despite similarity in name.)

The same physician reported that those who tested negative by the above test (about two-thirds of those who presumed they were affected by the disease according to their own questionnaire) actually suffered from other allergies, hypothyroidism, other infections, heavy metal toxicities (especially mercury from dental fillings and other sources) and various types of functional non-specific disorders.

His conservative conclusion was that there are probably some patients with intractable problems who should at least be tested for Candidiasis and if found positive, given a trial therapy appropriate, such as Ketoconazole.

Other physicians will place their suspected Candidiasis candidates on rather extensive, stringent diets sometimes lasting for a year or more along with various medicines of prescription and non-prescription natures.

I wish that I could report to you which approach is best — or perhaps that it is best not to take Candidiasis treatment at all — but I cannot do so. Like most of the alternative medicines described in this book, you and your physician will need to make up your own mind, especially after reading many books on the subject.

This I know: The treatment is generally safe in

whichever form it is offered to you, especially under a caring and knowledgeable physician interested in your welfare and in you as a personality, not a warehoused dollar source . It is generally low cost compared to other possible approaches. So, why not try it, if your doctor says to do so? It surely will not harm you.

I also know this: Virtually all Rheumatoid Disease victims are immunologically depressed — and Candidiasis grows well in such a deficient garden!

Many altenative/complementary physicians use diet and special medicines to treat against Candidiasis along with our treatment for Rheumatoid Disease. Those same physicians seem to show a higher success rate in halting the progress of RD.

You can obtain additional information from the Price-Pottenger Nutrition Foundation at 5871 El Cajon Blvd., San Diego, CA 92115. Send a self-addressed stamped legal size (large) envelope with five dollars and a list of physicians treating yeast problems will be sent to you.

Chapter IX
Nutritional Aspects of Rheumatoid Arthritis

A most valuable supplement with the use of our treatment protocol is proper nutrition. There have been many books written on the subject of nutrition for several generations as it relates to Rheumatoid Arthritis — and probably most of them are correct.

Some physicians and health oriented advisors will take the stand that nutrition alone can cure arthritis, and they also may be correct under certain conditions. It obviously happens with sufficient frequency for the truth to linger, but not with high enough frequency to convince all of us who have tragically become victims of the crippler.

What I believe happens is this: Factors that contribute to the precipitation of Rheumatoid Disease (RD) are genetic, stress, and weakening of the immunological system. Many people are under continuing stress, thus weakening their ability to fight off infection and Rheumatoid Arthritis. Several kinds of stress exist, including emotional, physical and nutritional.

Whenever we RD-prone folks ignore good nutritional habits over long periods, our bodies lose ability to produce the necessary fighting tools to ward off physical and emotional problems and also we lose the ability to repair tissues and organs properly under normal wear and tear.

If Rheumatoid Disease begins at this point, and if the individual returns to a good and proper diet at once, and if the individual knowingly or unknowingly reduces emotional stress, then I believe the regression of Rheumatoid Arthritis is much more likely without any further treatment — but not certain!

What is probably normal is that stress continues onward — we are unable to leave a particularly detested job, weighty family responsibilities seem unsolvable, children continue to perplex with persistent problems, husband or wife is a "suppressive personality", and so on.

Under such circumstances perhaps no amount of good nutritional habits will reverse the disease in genetically predisposed arthritics.

More than likely, the arthritic continues on with the same poor food habits of a lifetime, and so nutritional aspects are ignored in any case.

Perhaps either relief of stress or improved nutrition, or combinations of both "spontaneously" bring about remission of the disease, at least for the time being.

Usually initial resort is to the rheumatologist who, being trained in the traditional and "time-honored" "accepted" treatments (treating symptoms, not causes), first provides costly tests, presumably confirming the condition of arthritis. Then secondly aspirin is tried. When aspirin no longer helps (or becomes dangerous in quantities needed to suppress pain symptoms) he/she writes prescriptions for NSAIDS (non-steroidal anti-inflammatories). When these fail — and they eventually will — he/she advises use of dangerous gold shots which not only have damaging side-effects but in any case will not be effective — if at all — beyond thirty months. When this fails or proves too toxic for a patient to tolerate, penicillamine is used, and after that methotrexate. All of this will or will not accompany the increasing use of cortico-steroids in increasingly heavy dosages — and sickness rages onward!

Sadly, and unfortunately, some years ago rheumatologists voted to reverse this course, starting with the most damaging drug, methotrexate and working down to the least, aspirin. Such is their claim to "science based medicine" that this reversable protocol came about through a vote, not through scientific studies.

The peer group publication, *Clinics in Rheumatic Diseases* (ISBN: 0307-742x) published in December 1983 by W.B. Saunders & Co. is a scientific standard for evaluating clinical applications. It clearly shows that gold shots when subjected to standards of double-blind tests failed the pre-defined criteria by 1% but was accepted as a "safe and effective" treatment in any case. After thirty months, the "effectiveness" fails almost completely in any case. The studies, of course, do not dwell on the tremendous toxicity when using the drug, nor on the fact that after its use, the immunological system may be damaged.

The same publication presents the fact that there is absolutely no scientific evidence for the use of penicillamine, yet that is the substance often prescribed after gold fails. Penicillamine, of course, is also toxic and dangerous.

I believe that the chief advantage to use of penicillamine after use of gold is the fact that it is a chelator for the gold. A build up of gold in the bodily tissues contributes to increasing toxicities which add to the arthritic symptoms and burdens. The two symptoms — toxicity of gold and RD symptoms — appear to the patient as symptoms of progressive Rheumatoid Disease. When gold is no longer even marginally helpful, the physician, knowledgeably or otherwise, in resorting to penicillamine, chelates out (removes out) the toxic gold, thus giving the patient a sense of improvement as the symptoms due to toxicity of the gold is lifted from his/her tissues.

Of course, the Rheumatoid Disease rages onward.

When penicillamine fails, Methotrexate is often next, and it is a most dangerous and futile drug. I would challenge any physician to demonstrate that this drug, or any of those listed above will cure or bring about long-range remission of arthritis in any number of significant cases in quantities greater than the normal placebo effect of 30%! — which, of course, is not permanent remission via these traditional means.

It is most probable that had the rheumatologist instead concentrated on helping the patient to learn about and relieve stress and also to change dietary habits, the percentage of successes would have been greater than the placebo effect of 30%. This approach would have taken a great deal of extra time, at greater cost — or certainly lowered earning capacity for the physician. Sadly for our society, most physicians are taught by medical schools that instruct to treat symptoms, not causes, which results in the administering of drugs to relieve symptoms, not in searching out causes and teaching the patient to understand the stresses of his/her immediate environment. While this approach serves well pharmaceutical companies, and keeps patients returning to the physician's office, it cannot cure.

This process is rather hard on you and me.

It is difficult, if not impossible, to purchase the food that our bodies require from restaurants and quick-food franchises. While dieticians and corporate stock advisors explain how nutritious the local hamburger joint is, you and I as arthritics should be better educated and behave accordingly.

Like most folks I like mother's cooking best. She's deceased and I still like her recipes best. What you and I like to eat is what we've been conditioned to like from childhood, not of choice. Because we are able to make a choice, and because we always choose what we like best —mother's cooking — does not mean that we have exercised that free choice, or rather that we have determined our choices by our likes which were determined by our earlier conditioning — before we had a choice — which is no longer "free choice".

Since becoming a victim of arthritis I've read many books on nutrition, but I will not pretend to know what there is to know about the subject. Possibly one reason that the subject of proper nutrition is not taught in medical schools is that it is the most complex of medical subjects, requiring far more knowledge of the human biochemistry than modern day undergraduate medical schools can provide.

One good book on the subject is *Medical Applications of Clinical Nutrition* edited by Jeffrey Bland, Ph.D. and published by Keats Publishing Co. (ISBN: 087983-327-0).

Caution: This book is very stiff reading unless you've a medical background.

Maureen Salaman, former President of the National Health Federation, has studied the issue of nutrition in Cancer. Her book, *The Cancer Answer* (ISBN: 0-913087-00-9) is a remarkable summary of the chief tenets of good nutrition, not just for arthritics, but for everyone. The book can be purchased at Stratford Publishing, 1259 El Camino Real, Suite 1500, Menlo Park, CA 94025.

In *The Cancer Answer* excellent points are made that the closer we can get to eating as did our primitive forefathers, the healthier we shall be. After all, our bodies are the product of millions of years of evolution in conjunction with other organisms such as plants and animals. We have, through this joint-evolution, adapted, just as plants and other animals have adapted to our precursors.

"Normal" Diets vary worldwide and encompass for humans almost everything edible and safe, whether insect, mammal, cacti, fungi, eel, snake, fish, tuber . . .

In addition to our very early conditioning and the daily barrage of huxterism by food processing monopolies and fast food franchises, there is the fact that more and more polluting chemicals are being spread on our crops even as trace elements in their soil disappears. The food that looks so healthy in supermarkets may not be on laboratory analysis. So we, as arthritics, are faced with another problem: Where to get food that is wellness-forming?

Speaking of supermarkets, one health food article by specialists in biochemistry and nutrition starts out like this: There are two kinds of things that people place in their mouths and eat. One of these we shall call "food", and the other we shall call "non-food". We shall define "non-food" as every kind that is packaged, processed, frozen, refined, or otherwise changed from its natural form. This will include all canned goods, all dried fruits and vegetables, all sterilized and otherwise cooked foods that are then cooled and sold in supermarkets, all irradiated foods, and so on. Candies, gums, cakes, pies and such mixtures are also "non-food".

So what is left to be called "food"?

Well, fresh fruits and vegetables, nuts, whole grains and so on.

Incidentally, by this definition of "food", vitamins are not foods, as they are the result of having been processed or synthesized.

The point is that "food" is nature's complete package container that has not only a lot of nutritional elements that we need and know about, but also a lot of food elements that we need and don't know about, particularly trace minerals and compounds that our body will utilize for processes unknown. Processing nature's package for convenience and long shelf life destroys necessary compounds or eliminates trace elements.

Each of us was created uniquely and endowed genetically different, which means that each of us has different nutritional requirements in addition to a commonalty of nutritional requirements. Anyone who tells you that you need so and so in certain amounts to be healthy is probably mistaken, just as the standard minimum daily requirements of vitamins and minerals when applied to the individual are usually mistaken. The reason that the minimum daily requirements as to daily amount required is usually wrong is because such figures represent averages of groups of people, not unique individual requisites for you. Some folks require far, far more Vitamin D than others, and can tolerate enough that would poison others. Whenever a physician or know-it-all academician tells you that you <u>must</u> or <u>must not</u> take a certain amount of a vitamin or mineral each day to be healthy, in the absence of specific information about you, he/she is ignorant of individual differences and how the minimum daily requirements were ascertained. For the most part, the standards of minimum daily requirements for vitamins and minerals were established as <u>lower</u> boundary to prevent disease states, like scurvy, **not** to define quantities required to furnish individualized wellness!

Neither can anyone tell you exactly what foods to eat, and how much, except in special circumstances where disease states are to be prevented, and certain requirements are well known outside of your individuality. Consider vitamin C, for example. As you are probably aware, there has been much controversy over the usage of vitamin C in larger or smaller quantities. Only certain mammals besides man are incapable of producing their own vitamin C. Did you ever wonder how so many animals, like dogs and cats, can eat garbage and disease-ridden foods and remain healthy? It is because God has found in his wisdom that their bodies shall produce the chemicals required to fight off infection and poisons, and vitamin C is a requisite part of that system.

As I will cover later, Robert F. Cathcart, M.D., one of our former referral physicians, has shown that each individual, at different times during the day, and on differing days, requires differing amounts of vitamin C to handle stress, disease and other physiological problems.

It becomes clearer with the study of various dietary recommendations, that Maureen Salaman's recommendations are probably one of the best synthesis in the dietary field, and should be read by all lay people.

Different people require different things, and they require different things at different times. As people grow, mature, and become old, they require differing quantities and different things. Different disease states require differing quantities. The field of nutrition and nutritional supplements is indeed complex — too complex for simplistic answers.

What is wrong with our diets is easier to answer: We Americans consume 18 percent of our calories as refined sugar which has no vitamins or minerals necessary for metabolism. We consume another 18 percent of our calories in the form of refined, enriched white flour which is nutritionally deficient in about 28 essential nutrients, including vitamin B[6].

From the Price-Pottenger Nutrition Foundation, see their excellent *Nourishing Traditions* a cookbook by Sally Fallon, Ph.D. and Pat Connelly.

There are no easy answers to nutrition. You must solve the problems yourself. You must find the best fresh fruit and vegetables possible, and you should probably supplement your diet in ways that are guided by the best nutritionally oriented physician possible. Additionally you should read books about the nutritional aspects of arthritis.

Having stated some of the general principles that apply,

and my personal conclusions, I now go on to the Foundation's treatment protocol respecting nutrition.

Having first had the Foundation treatment for Rheumatoid Disease, and having halted disease progress, I was able to maintain my wellness state for but two to three months at a time. Our treatment says to take a trial dosage every six months to learn if one again has the Herxheimer, indicating renewal of the disease. If so, one is to then take the full six week treatment. I found that I was taking the medicine every two to three months, and from time to time suffering for an evening or so with a severe Herxheimer reaction.

Note that the Herxheimer reaction lasted me, during these trial periods, but an evening or so during which I was terribly sick, to the point where I cared less if the world turned or not. But the next morning I would feel absolutely great again, and ready to tackle the lions of this world. As a precautionary measure, of course, I would complete the full treatment for six weeks.

I also received letters and talked to people having the same repeat cycle. As earlier reported, we learned from a research pharmacologist that metabolization of Metronidazole required good intestinal microflora, and I therefore supplemented with *Lactobacilus acidophilus*, but that obviously was not the complete answer. To be cured meant to me not to have return of disease. Physicians will accept a "cure" of tonsillitis, and call its return as "another infection" which was not good enough for me with a disease that might still lead to crippling each time it returned.

We arthritics will not be satisfied with two to three months halt in disease progress, although that is infinitely better than no halt at all.

And so, during those early Foundation days we continued our search for a better answer for ourselves, in addition to pushing to the limit of our resources various University research.

Some of our referral physicians constantly spoke to us about the importance of diet, which we ignored, as some of our other physicians who are not diet oriented still do.

I, like you, was severely conditioned by mother's cooking. I also believed the physician who was generally unlearned respecting nutrition, but rather prescribed pills and shots for everything — the symptomatic approach — treat symptoms and ignore the cause! Usually their doggerel is that "your present diet furnishes you with all necessary vitamins and minerals."

False!

At last I paid attention to the diet requirements for arthritics. The principles are quite simple. The intestinal track must have acidity (hydrochloric acid) to properly utilize food and prevent overgrowth of "bad-guys" microflora. Other bodily tissues should be slightly basic, rather than acidic. A simple test developed by Carl Reich, M.D. of Canada using pH litmus paper told me that my saliva was exceedingly acidic, whereas testing of other healthy people, children and friends, found that their saliva was alkaline.

My new goal: To eat proper foods so that the saliva test would become alkaline, rather than acidic. It took me two years — mostly of procrastinating (remember my mother's early conditioning) — before I turned this test about, and also sustained permanency in relief from the arthritic condition!

To eat properly at last, I followed Gus Prosch's, Jr.,

M.D. advice. He was also a specialist in clinical nutrition as well as one of our former referral physicians.

His recommendations follow shortly.

Candidiasis diet is more restrictive than a general arthritic diet, and should probably be followed first. Prosch uses many products. There are other commercial products for Candidiasis, but aside from the Candidiasis factor, Prosch, in speaking before our Second Annual Medical Convention, continued with:

I would like to discuss the importance of diet, nutrition and vitamin and mineral supplementation in Rheumatoid Disease patients. Many different opinions and conclusions among most physicians today are fairly rampant and many doctors do not believe this subject is important, so I'm going to tell you about my beliefs and observations as to how and why I treat my patients, but I want to stress that these methods are my own opinions and not those of The Rheumatoid Disease Foundation.

In my observations and research there are several things that to me stand out to be quite significant in most patients with Rheumatoid Disease.

1. The great majority of Rheumatoid Disease patient's body fluids are too acid in nature.

2. The great majority of these patients show signs and symptoms of a deficiency in free or ionic calcium.

3. Most Rheumatoid Disease patients eat margarine instead of butter and they demonstrate a lack of Vitamin A and natural D[3] plus severe deficiencies of the essential fatty acids.

4. Diet in Rheumatoid Disease does help control the severity of the symptoms.

5. Vitamin and mineral supplementations help shorten the recovery time by strengthening the immune

78

system.

In studying the nutrition status and diet of Rheumatoid Disease patients, I made three observations that have caused me to look deeper into this subject.

1. I observed that many patients who are blood-related to arthritic patients do not develop any arthritis especially when different dietary habits were followed.

2. I observed that often-times arthritic patients exhibited slight to significant improvement when self-administered home and folk remedies were taken, like alfalfa tablets, bone meal tablets, cod liver oil, vinegar with honey, peanut oil, . . . or cherries.

3. I observed that some arthritic patients are more susceptible to getting reinfected after being treated with the medication that apparently eliminated the offending organisms.

I found by checking the acidity of saliva and urine of arthritic patients, that the great majority were considerably more acid than normal and I concluded that an alkaline diet could only benefit these patients.

I also found by careful observation that Rheumatoid Disease patients more often than normal exhibited certain physical signs during the physical examination. To summarize these signs, they are as follows:

1. Longitudinal ridges and increased opaqueness in fingernails.

2. Mild to moderate tenderness with strong palpation of the soleus or trapezius muscles.

3. Generalized slight increase in deep tendon reflexes.

4. Generalized irritability of skeletal muscles to percussion.

5. Acid saliva of pH 4.5 to 6.5.

6. Slight to severe coating on the tongue.

Many of these signs are related to calcium metabolism in the body and most arthritic patients drink 2% or low fat milk and eat margarine instead of butter.

The previously mentioned physical signs demonstrate strong evidence of free or ionic calcium deficiency as well as a deficiency of Vitamin A and D[3] which is natural Vitamin D. Blood calcium studies are misleading as they measure the ionic calcium as well as calcium bound to proteins. Whereas normal body fluids ideally are slightly alkaline as opposed to acid, and I believe the one primary cause of the deficiency in Rheumatoid Disease patients of the ionic calcium which in itself is very alkaline.

An even more important cause of this acidity is due to the diet and nutritional habits of these arthritic patients. Most cellular mechanisms of the body and particularly those involving the use of ionized minerals such as the secretory glands, nerve function processes and muscle contraction, etc. proceed best in a mildly alkaline state. For this reason a diet consisting of high alkaline foods should be consumed, combined with the avoidance of acid forming foods. Alkaline high are potassium, calcium, magnesium and sodium. Acid forming foods are those which are high in one or more of four elements: phosphorus, sulphur and chlorine. The diet used to treat and prevent development of Rheumatoid Diseases should definitely avoid as much as possible the following foods. All processed and most canned foods should be avoided along with caffeine, sugar in all it's forms, as well as the simple carbohydrate foods that quickly upon digestion turn into sugar, like white flour foods, crackers, many cereals, macaroni (pasta foods) white rice and corn products. Ideally nicotine and alcohol should be avoided, along with any sweets, candy, soft drinks, pastries and desserts. The "nightshade plants" (foods containing solanines) such as white potatoes, tomatoes, egg plant and garden peppers should be avoided. (Robert Bingham, M.D. states that about 1/3 of arthritics are affected by solanines:Ed.).

As a rule, most protein foods tend to be acid forming since they contain phosphorus and sulfur. Animal sources of protein — lean meat (beef, lamb, veal) poultry, fish and eggs — are definitely in this category. With the exception of shrimp, most sea food is extremely acid forming. These foods must not be avoided however in the diet, as they provide the building blocks for all body functions and processes. Therefore one of these proteins should be eaten with each meal. Pork meats should be limited however. Just try not to eat an entire meal consisting of protein foods, but balance these foods with alkaline forming foods. Ideally your breakfast should always consist of some high protein foods, balanced with whole milk, fruit juices, etc. Also remember to cook protein foods at low temperatures, as enzymes and trace minerals are reduced with excessive heat and no foods should be eaten that have been deep fried.

Avoid processed and hydrogenated, or "hardened" oils and fats. Most margarines, peanut butters, restaurant prepared french fries and potato or corn chips are prepared with hardened oils. Sweet cream butter is best and use "cold pressed" vegetable oils or "Pam" for home cooking. (Pam once contained olive oil, but no longer. Instead, use Mazola Pro Chef, but be sure to read the labels as there is one kind that uses olive oil, and another in the same can and with the same label, that does not. Ed.) Also watch those high calorie salad dressings. Most fats and fatty foods (butter, oils, sausages, bacon, etc.) are neutral *in their acid-alkaline content but they greatly contribute to excessive weight gain which severely complicates arthritis. Therefore, it would be wise to limit all oily, greasy, fried, fatty foods if one tends to be overweight.* (According to Ray Peat, Ph.D. and Jane Heimlich, coconut oil is excellent for many reasons. Ed.)

Most all vegetables (except corn) are highly alkaline in nature and should be emphasized in the eating program. Salad vegetables are excellent and should be eaten daily. All other vegetables are very good and when "Wok" cooked or stir fried in cold pressed vegetable oil are even better.

Fresh vegetable juices (not canned) are nearly perfect and should be part of the diet. It is important to prepare and serve as many foods in their raw and natural state as possible.

All fruits and fruit juices (excepting cranberries, plums and prunes) are alkaline forming and are good to "munch" on.

Whole milk is one of the best alkaline forming foods due to its high calcium content. Raw certified whole milk is much preferable if you can find it. (available in Arizona, California, Georgia: Ed.) *At least two glasses of whole milk should be taken each day and use butter instead of margarine. Plain yogurt is an excellent alkalinizing food and not only is easy to digest, but tastes great when mixed with fresh fruit such as raisins, dates, dried figs and apricots. It also makes excellent munching foods.*

This diet will change one's system to be more alkaline as it should be.

Concerning vitamin and mineral supplementation, the most important point to consider here is to correct the free calcium deficiency present in most arthritics. This requires much larger amounts of vitamin A and D in their natural form than what is usually recommended by the "Recommended Daily Allowances" tables.

The synthetic Vitamin A and D[2] preparations on the market simply do not work. Synthetic Vitamin D[2] does increase the calcium absorption from the small intestine but seems to be totally inadequate in regulating the use of the calcium and especially calcium excretion by the kidneys. The only preparation I have found that is adequate is the natural D[3] which is found in fish liver oils. Therefore I recommend Norwegian Cod Liver Oil as the ideal which seems to be even better than cod liver oil capsules. It is easily taken when mixed with some orange juice and stirred rapidly. The preparation I recommend is plain Norwegian Cod Liver Oil liquid which contains 10,000 units of Vitamin A and 1000 units of Vitamin D per teaspoon. I recommend that patients take two teaspoons on arising each morning and two teaspoons at bedtime. This preparation can be found in most health food stores and should be taken for at least four months, then the dosage should be cut in half.

I explain to the patients not to fear any Vitamin A or D toxicity with this dosage as it is less than 1/3 the toxicity level that has been reported in the literature. If the patient absolutely cannot take the liquid, they can usually find capsules at a health food store which will provide approximately 4,000 units of Vitamin D daily.

I also explain that exposure to sunshine for at least 20 minutes each week will activate the Vitamin D.

Concerning the calcium preparations I have found that none of the available inorganic calcium preparations are effective. I discovered that organic bone meal tablets (3-4 per day) work better than other calcium preparations but I continued to have reservations. Recently I located a calcium preparation which seems to work ideally. It is the naturally occurring calcium in plants. I prescribe 500 mg. This compound is Calcium Orotate (500 mg 4 times daily).

This calcium preparation also seems to enhance the ability of the body to use and metabolize other forms of calcium ingested.

I also prescribe 500 mg of Magnesium Orotate twice daily to balance the calcium/magnesium ratio. The above calcium preparation is also excellent for osteoporosis and it greatly strengthens the bone and cartilage structures in the body.

Concerning other vitamins for arthritic patients, I recommend as an ideal supplemental program the following:

a. Vitamin B Complex, two to three "Stress" B vitamins daily in divided doses. (These should contain 50-75 mg of each B vitamin).

b. Vitamin C, two to three grams daily in divided doses.

c. Zinc Orotate, 500 mg one to two tablets on an empty stomach.

d. Selenium, 250 micrograms daily as yeast selenium.

e. B-Carotene, 25,000 units daily.

f. Vitamin E, 400 units daily.

The above vitamin and mineral supplementations will not only help the patient's arthritis by stimulating the immune response system but will play an important role in counteracting the aging process as well as acting as a deterrent to some forms of cancer since many of these preparations act as free radical and peroxide scavengers in the body.

With painful hands and feet, I recommend in addition

100 mg Vitamin B[6], 4 times daily. This is also good for Carpal Tunnel Syndrome.

With Neuralgia I suggest 500 mg niaciniamide 4 times daily.

Another very important supplement that I find is necessary in all patients with Rheumatoid Disease is essential fatty acids.

Before going into this part, let me digress a moment and discuss some vital information about our number one killer today — coronary artery disease. We have been told the past 30 years that it's our cholesterol intake that causes this hardening of the arteries and coronary artery disease. This is simply not so and let me explain why and I think you will agree with me.

Before 1900 "heart attacks" were hardly known and the first recognized account of this disease in the medical literature was published in 1912. The diets of Americans at that time consisted of high cholesterol foods such as butter, eggs, lard, sowbelly and red meats rich in saturated fats, yet heart attacks were so rare that most U.S. doctors didn't even know what they were.

In the 1920's hydrogenated oils and processed foods were introduced into our society. The food companies added hydrogen to margarines, corn and other cooking oils to make them more solid or hard.

At this time the food companies began processing foods so that they would last a long time on the shelves. By removing all the essential fatty acids, the foods would not turn rancid or spoil. The food companies remove the fatty acids from all our cereal and grain foods such as wheat, oats, rye, barley, corn, etc. Americans living before the 1920's who didn't have heart attacks ate unprocessed foods and all their grains and cereal foods were whole ground and contained the essential fatty acids necessary to maintain good health.

Some of the dietary cholesterol we eat is absorbed into our system but our body primarily manufactures it's own cholesterol. The key to hardening of the arteries and heart attacks therefore is to learn why our bodies do not use the cholesterol properly that our own body manufactures. I've known for years that cholesterol in our diet cannot be the major cause of heart attacks because the Iceland Eskimos in their diet take in 10 times more cholesterol than we do, yet they develop hardening of the arteries or heart attacks much, much less frequently than we Americans who eat much less cholesterol. The two factors involved here are: (1) the Eskimos eat no hydrogenated oils, and (2) they eat large amounts of non-farmed, cold water fish which have a high content of the essential fatty acids. Give these Eskimos hydrogenated oils and processed foods and they begin developing heart attacks like we do.

Another example, in World War II when the Germans overran Norway, the Norwegians had a very high incidence of heart attacks, cancer and schizophrenia. The Germans took away all the margarines and the incidence of heart attacks, cancer and schizophrenia dropped significantly. When the Germans left and the Norwegians resumed eating their margarines, these diseases increased again.

Unfortunately, in America, we are developing hardening of the arteries faster today and at an earlier age than ever before. In the Korean War, autopsies performed on 18 to 23 year old casualties showed 30% had advanced hardening of the arteries. Years later, in the Vietnamese War, autopsies showed that 60% of the casualties had this condition. And every day now we hear of young men in their twenties having heart attacks. So our society is developing this serious condition at earlier ages and our society is getting more hydrogenated oils and less essential fatty acids than ever before.

Recent research is showing that the hydrogenated oils actually block the way our bodies use our cholesterol. Also, without the essential fatty acids, our bodies cannot use cholesterol properly and we develop an imbalance in certain chemicals called prostaglandins that can help cause or prevent heart attacks.

What can you do for yourself and your family to help prevent the development of hardening of the arteries and heart attacks?

First of all, get all hydrogenated oils out of your house such as found in margarines, cooking oils and all deep fried foods like donuts, french fries, potato chips and corn chips. Most desserts like cookies, pies and cakes are loaded with hydrogenated oils. You can use instead cold pressed oils if "cold pressed" is written on the label.

Second, we all must increase the good fatty acids in our diets by eating non-farmed, cold water ocean fish 3-4 times weekly, like salmon, mackerel, herring, sardines, tuna and codfish.

We should also eat at least one tablespoon of virgin olive oil daily. (Not "pure" olive oil.) It is good mixed with salads. Also walnuts are very high in these necessary fatty acids. And we should totally avoid all processed breads and flour products such as white breads, crackers, macaroni, spaghetti and pasta foods. One hundred percent whole wheat or whole grain breads are okay if the label says 100% whole grain.

There are 3 main essential fatty acids we all need for

proper functioning of all cellular metabolism and to keep the proper balance of our good and bad prostaglandins. These fatty acids we all need for proper functioning of all cellular metabolism and to keep the proper balance of our good and bad prostaglandins. These fatty acids are Eicosapentanoic and Docosahexanoic acids and our bodies can manufacture Gamma-Linolenic acid from Cis-Linoleic acid under normal conditions. However, there is an enzyme called Delta-6-De-Saturase that must be present to convert the Cis-Linoleic acid to Gamma Linolenic acid. This enzyme is blocked when we take in hydrogenated oils or when there is a deficiency of Vitamin C, B[6], B[3] or Magnesium and Zinc to name a few.

Gamma-Linolenic acid is found naturally in sufficient amounts in human breast milk and Oil of Evening Primrose seeds. By giving patients Evening Primrose Oil itself, we don't have to worry about converting the Cis-Linoleic to the Gamma-Linolenic acid.

Without the Gamma-Linolenic acid balance in the body, an excess of arachidonic acid is made which causes an excess amount of Leukotrienes to be manufactured and these chemicals are up to 500 times more potent than histamines in inflammatory reactions. The Gamma-linolenic acid is absolutely mandatory to suppress the inflammatory processes that are so prevalent in these diseases.

So I give all Rheumatoid Disease patients salmon oil and Evening Primrose Oil capsules to be sure that these necessary fatty acids are available to the body. This reduces inflammation and helps prevent hardening of the arteries at the same time. I give 4-6 capsules of each daily for build-up in the body.

You must be very careful about the Evening Primrose

88

Oil that is prescribed as it is not available in the U.S. and must come from England. I would estimate that 80% of Evening of Primrose Oil sold in the U.S. today is nothing more than soy bean oil mis-labeled as Evening Primrose Oil.

I know some physicians will not agree with me about some of this information, but I am getting good to excellent results in about 80% of my patients. I only hope this talk will inspire physicians hearing this lecture or others who may hear a copy of the tape to treat their patients properly so they will also get excellent results in relieving the pain and agony of their arthritic patients.

Many of our physicians recognize the importance of diet in getting and staying well. While they will often argue over fine points, they do not disagree on the major. For example, where Gus Prosch, M.D. recommends whole milk, because of its very high calcium content, John Baron, D.O. our Foundation Chairman, states that the "calcium bioavailability in milk is less than 15%." Homogenized milk contains xanthine oxidase, an enzyme not found in significant quantity in human milk, which contributes greatly to atherosclerosis in the young. The primary problem, according to Dr. Baron, is that cow's milk, as a food, has been changed so greatly over the years by processing it into stable shelf life, that it is almost unrecognizable as a natural, nutritional, life-supporting material for humans. Homogenized milk is probably the worst, as the process of homogenizing breaks fat globules so that xanthine oxidase, instead of passing through as would be normal, provides very tiny particles that prove destructive by attacking the lining of our circulatory system (intima) beginning a pitting that starts the atherosclerotic process.

Neither Prosch nor Baron would disagree on the dangers of xanthine oxidase in homogenized milk or the desirability of whole, certified, raw milk as opposed to pasteurized milk.

For generations children and adults have been conditioned to believe in the impeccability of the grocer's milk — the perfect food, some have propagandized. Did you know that we Americans subsidize the Dairy Industry to the amount of $2,000,000 per year, and that such a powerful monopoly thus formed has entrenched itself into the food-agriculture system so that truth must be sought in other than public forums?

The historical and persistent efforts to drive out certified, whole milk as sold by Alta-Dena Diaries of California is an excellent example on how we have permitted good nutrition to be prosecuted while believing the dollar-hungry propagandist. I recommend reading *The Milk of Human Kindness is Not Pasteurized* by one of our former referral physicians, William Campbell Douglass, M.D.

But to get back to my personal saga: at last I followed Dr. Gus Prosch's advice, deliberately changing my dietary habits. I never liked salads, derogatorily calling them "rabbit food". I learned to like them, as well as to decrease my consumption of acid forming foods such as red meats (hamburger). I increased fresh fruits and vegetables and whole grains and nuts.

Lo!

The diet worked. I did turn about the saliva test from acidic to basic. Had I not been so blind — and yes, stubborn — I could have done that two years earlier and saved a lot of pain and pill taking.

I haven't taken any medicine listed on our treatment

90

protocol for thirty-one years (1999). You must admit that is a remarkable time period compared against the two to three month cycle I was forced to accept earlier!

Most family physicians, though quite well-meaning, and otherwise well trained in medicine, do not know enough about nutrition to advise you properly. It is doubtful that many dieticians, although college trained, are capable of doing so either. I say this knowing full well that there is bound to be considerable response against my attitude. But consider: graduate, licensed dieticians are responsible for the most part for the nutritionless foods given to patients in hospitals, and which is clearly the source of many in-hospital deaths due to malnutrition. There is no way of knowing how many sick patients have died unnecessarily because of starvation when they most needed fresh fruits and vegetables because of surgical stress.

If you are not already aware of the great conflict that exists between those who represent "establishment" medicine and those who represent "alternative" medicines, then you should become acquainted with it. In recent years there has been a flood of new discoveries in the fields of nutrition and use of food supplements. Amongst legitimate discoveries, quack advertisements abound. Congressional investigations as well as advocates of freedom of choice in medicine are in conflict, because of the inability to separate "good guys" from "bad guys". Sadly, usually those with the most financial clout are able to make the greatest impact on the news media, causing the general public to believe that the good-guys are really the bad-guys, and vice versa. They use the emotional button of "quack" to attach to anyone and anything that is not paid for, owned and controlled by the pharmaceutical and food/agricultural monopolies. Having control of so many bucks, and consequently such heavy political and news-media clout, these vested interests can gain the ears and eyes, hands and feet of all of the major Federal and State agencies to go after those they deem contrary to their financial stake.

The process is relatively simple: Through local medical associations, go after physicians who do not use the same treatments that everyone else uses. Often censure, temporary suspension or revocation of licenses result — as is near certain when a physician chooses to use alternative medicines instead of treatments that are doomed to failure at the start. If temporary revocation results, insurance companies withdraw insurance. Without insurance, a physician can no longer have hospital privileges. Such an experience is frequent throughout the United States today, and physician after physician is being asked to defend themselves and their procedures because they dare to try to help a patient, rather than to use already doomed medical practices.

Similarly, various products are ripped from health food stores through action by the FDA. Often various governmental and private organizations band together under the banner of "Remove Quackery", and never does the public dream that the real quacks are those who are instigators of the actions.

Unfortunately for us, there are real "quacks" out there who do rip off money under false pretenses or who use fraudulent schemes and sell worthless products falsely advertised, and we certainly need protection against these — so I cannot fault the purpose of it all.

What I do fault is the inability to discriminate between the good guy and the bad guy, and the indiscriminate labeling of everything that is different from what is already in practice and found ineffective.

This book was not written to expose fraudulent expose'. Instead, I refer the reader to several publications that can be found online where may also be found nutritional advice of high quality, clinical and research findings involving alternative medicines and the truth about our threat against freedom of choice in medicine:

There is much that is good in the idea of assuring that we are not harmed, but in practice, the whole issue is subverted by so many extraneous or expeditious considerations for a particular medical treatment that what is good is often screened out, and what is bad continues to dominate the "establishment" field of medical practice. Consider, for example, the approval of such drugs as gold, penicillamine, methotrexate and long-term cortico-steroids in the treatment of arthritics. All have passed the FDA's "safe" and "effective" criteria, yet each in their own way are often more damaging than the disease it purports to relieve symptomatically.

On the other hand, those who administer alternative treatments such as EDTA Chelation Therapy (more on this later), DMSO treatment, and various nutritional supplemental programs are harassed and hounded by local medical associations, yet all are known to be effective for various kinds of diseases and all are eminently safe when compared against those already so-called "proved".

As otherwise responsible American citizens, you and I permit what amounts to buffoonery. See, for example, *Racketeering In Medicine: The Suppression of Alternatives* by James P. Carter, Ph.D., Dr. P.H.

There is already a remarkable amount of literature written on the false illusion presented by minimum vitamin and mineral daily requirements. Among all of the legitimate complaints is the fact that no matter how scientifically accurate the minimum vitamin and mineral standards are performed, they still represent a single number that stands for "averages" of groups of animals or people. It does not reflect either yours or my genetic make-up, and we are all different, as different as the size of leaves on a tree. Those sizes, we all know, vary from very tiny to very large, very wide to very thin, very venous to lacking in many veins, and so on.

The body's requirement for Vitamin C, for example, varies from person to person, day to day, sickness to sickness, and cannot be determined by means of an "average" figure, or by any other single number. Both two time Nobel Prize winner Linus D. Pauling, Ph.D. and Robert Cathcart, M.D. (one of our former referral physicians) have shown this statement to be true beyond reproach. More on Cathcart's work later.

You can pay for detailed analysis of your biochemistry (within the state-of-the-art) to determine some of your biochemical needs. Such analysis when provided by competent and specialized laboratories will give your physician great insight as to what you lack for the moment. It is possible that such insight will help to correct that lack.

Even such a straightforward approach can be costly, and some physicians try to circumvent that cost by using a means that I think is an absurdity and, perhaps, plays on the gullibility of their patient, if not displaying their own naivete'.

I have been tested by physicians who take a blood sample and send it off to a laboratory where a computer analysis is mailed back purporting to know not only the state of my vitamin and mineral deficiencies, but also presenting me with several dozen sheets of computerized output that presumably analyzes all of my nutritional needs, and tells me what I should take to remedy the situation presumed to be wrong.

These recommendations, based on single blood and/ or hair tests, are nonsense, and, if anything, should be labeled as nutritional quackery, in my opinion.

Firstly, there is no adjunctive measure of tissue supplies or the rates at which I am losing or gaining various vitamins and minerals from the body. High measures within blood, for example, could easily mean that my body is flushing valuable ingredients out of tissues, where they are needed. Hair samples (properly done) tell other things about processes. When considered, and watched over a period of time, coupled with patient history, and physician knowledge of the history, such tests can be highly useful and inexpensive when compared against the cost of purchasing follow-through bio-chemical analysis of various enzyme reactions — although these tests might also be required for proper evaluation.

A doctor who, however, simply sends in the blood, and mails you the computer output is either ignorant of nutritional processes or is taking an easy route to get more money from your pocketbook, in my opinion.

If statistical averages are relatively meaningless for establishing our individual vitamin and mineral needs, then why isn't it equally meaningless when interpreting automated computer analyses from isolated blood samples?

As I've already stated, the subject of nutritional needs and vitamin and mineral needs is probably the most complex of medical subjects. Physicians for the most part know little about this biochemical realm. They are simply not taught it in undergraduate medical school and probably have not studied it intensively since graduating.

There's little question that we arthritics do have vitamin and mineral deficiencies, but whether they stem from upset biochemistries, inability to absorb nutritients, liver damage from cancer or infection, lack of appropriate nutritients, ancillary disease states, or what have you, is a mighty tangled web to unweave. Most people do not have sufficient income to pay for all of the analyses and "expert" help required to do the untangling — and so, for the most part, but certainly with a specialist's help, we need to begin the untangling ourselves.

Like all the other treatments I recommend, it will be up to you to separate out who can help you and who cannot, for more than knowledge is involved in a patient/ physician relationship — also trust and faith and convenience and cost.

The body has many "fail-safe" biochemical systems that allow chemical pathways to follow down alternate chains. Certain reactions will take place, producing certain end products not normal to the body, if certain chemicals are missing but others are present. A good analogy is that which happens to food plants. If certain minerals are not available in the soil, but others are, the plant may very well take up the secondary metals. The plant will then not be as nutritious, but it will have survived — which is apparently the purpose behind so many alternate pathways.

Where there is most complexity there is also the most confusion, especially when a subject is not well understood. There are a lot of publications and "advice" on the subject of nutrition. Unfortunately not all authors, specialists, Authorities, physicians, scientists, et al. always agree.

There are general principles to be understood and applied, and that is what you must do to begin learning for yourself. Dr. Prosch's talk, quoted herein, is a good beginning.

There is some danger in taking any one adviser for literal truth, although they may very well be telling it right for your purposes. One example suffices: Our treatment protocol calls for sometime and possible use of Copper Ions as designed and tested by one of our former referral physicians, Seldon Nelson, D.O. Properly speaking, these are food supplements rather than medicines, and are generally safe. We know that most arthritics have had tests leading to the conclusion that they lack copper.

An easy presumption is that arthritics should be furnished with copper supplements. Running out to the health food store for copper chelates will not necessarily turn the trick because: (1) you may lack the copper because of an inability to receive it in the correct compounds, (2) you have an inability to absorb it, (3) you have related chemical reactions that are the cause of the lack, (4) copper supplements may not apply to you at all, (5) other reasons known and unknown.

Copper is also antagonistic to zinc, and zinc to copper when taken simultaneously. Too much of one in the human system may drive out the other, and vice versa. By increasing either in the wrong dosages, ratios of copper to zinc are disturbed. This might be exactly the opposite of what you want to happen.

If I can make such a big issue out of such a simple thing as daily requirements for copper, think of how complex it gets when we add in all human nutritional requirements and their interactions!

I do not pretend to be any kind of expert, Authority or specialist in this field and, like you, I just try to learn what I can to help along my own needs toward wellness. I shan't beg the issue further.

When you do read books, and listen to the experts, keep the simple principle in mind that there is more to nutrition than meets the stomach, so to speak!

One aspect of nutrition is very important for arthritics to understand, which is that of "free radical scavengers" as will be discussed later under the subject of Chelation Therapy. Arthritics through inflammatory processes, generate a great deal of free radicals, which in turn create other damaging processes that often permanently damage our organs and tissues.

Those vitamins that are natural "scavengers" are known as "antioxidants" and they are Vitamins A, C, E, B[1], B[5], B[6]; and the amino acid L-Cysteine; the food antioxidants BHT and BHA; the minerals selenium and zinc.

Foods that contain these ingredients may be advantageous to an arthritic. More than that, and under careful selection, these antioxidants can individually and in various combinations be used to help reduce the inflammatory load.

Free radicals are atoms or molecules with an unpaired electron. These are chemically reactive entities that are produced in the normal course of our daily metabolism. We break-down peroxidized fats in the body by exposure to radiation and by ozone interactions with lipids (fats), the attack of oxidizing agents on fatty acids, particularly those that are unsaturated (see Prosch's comments on saturated versus unsaturated fats presented earlier), and so on.

Free radicals are major sources of damage causing aging (cross-linking of molecules), cardiovascular disease and cancer.

Free radical scavengers are molecules that can block free radical reactions. Antioxidants combine with free radicals, stopping their adverse actions.

Free radicals, by the way, are absolutely essential within the immunological system, under controlled conditions, for the purpose of killing germs that cause diseases, and they assist in neutralizing foreign invaders.

It is the balance between free radicals and antioxidants that gets out of kilter, for many and various reasons in an arthritic and thereby creates excessive inflammatory responses and consequent damage.

Vitamin E is a particularly excellent antioxidant. However, read the label. If it states that the contents are "esterfied", don't purchase it. The reason is this: When natural Vitamin E is packaged, it will be unstable unless stabilized for extra shelf life. Many scientists will tell you that the esterfied Vitamin E is as good as the unesterfied, but according to Dr. Gus Prosch, Jr., letters received by him from pharmaceutical companies indicate that the esterfied Vitamin E has no antioxidant properties.

Since the major purpose for taking the Vitamin E is to take advantage of its antioxidant properties, the purchase seems rather wasted.

Dr. Prosch purchases his Vitamin E for patients from A.C. Grace Company. This might be the only source of unesterfied Vitamin E in the U.S.

Dr. Prosch also mentioned in his talk the use of Evening of Primrose Oil for decrease of the inflammatory responses due to having consumed the wrong oils and fats in our general diet. Apparently there is no FDA control over the labeling of this product as to what shall be called "Primrose" oil, and so many, — apparently the majority of nutritional sales — sell "Primrose Oil" that is actually soybean oil packaged under that name. Soybean oil is useless for the purposes indicated, and a fraud when so packaged. A company that can provide genuine Primrose Oil is Bio-Tech and also it can be purchased as Efamol and Nature's Way, two acceptable brands available at most health food stores.

As you hopefully have noted, the whole field of nutrition is fraught with pitfalls of every kind that need much study and circumspectful analysis when applied to you and me.

Chapter X
Chelation Therapy

Chelation Therapy is one of the most effective supplementary treatments for Rheumatoid Diseases, including Rheumatoid Arthritis. It is a treatment of the future available for moderate to low cost now. It is the only treatment with which I am familiar given to the physician by him/herself and administered to his/her loved ones on a routine and often periodic basis.

Chelation Therapy has a definite place in the ridding of free-radicals that cause inflammation. It performs other duties that permit functioning for health, and because it operates at a level that is basic for the health of individual cells, Chelation Therapy also applies to and is indicated for virtually every disease and disease state. Oxygen atoms and other chemicals within the body are attracted to other compounds and atoms. The molecules and atoms that "seek" out, or have a very strong affinity for, other compounds and atoms are called "free radicals". Excessive free radicals damage tissues and promote cartilage decomposition and many other cascading problems for organs, systems and tissues generally.

Chelation Therapy is not an accepted process by the general medical establishment. In some few states, medical boards have closed down or prosecuted physicians who practice Chelation Therapy. These State Medical Boards for the most part consist of well-meaning physicians who are concerned with yours and my welfare (and their own pocketbooks in some cases), but who know absolutely nothing about the therapy, other than what they've read that was written by others who know nothing about it.

Virtually every article written against Chelation Therapy and printed in "respectable" journals has been written by a physician or researcher who has assumed the mantle of Authority, yet has absolutely no knowledge of it.

Critics of Chelation Therapy have never used it on themselves, nor their loved ones, nor on their patients, nor have they read the voluminous literature that has been compiled by various physicians and scientists who are members of the American College of Advancement in Medicine (ACAM), an organization dedicated to the practice of Chelation Therapy and to further research of it.

Cypher, Inc. of Ohio, which consisted of a group of physicians and Ph.Ds. They funded unpublished clinical research on the use of Chelation Therapy from clinical data gathered over the past fifteen years involving 20,000 patients. Statistical evaluations were performed by an independent organization, free from all bias.

Their study unequivocally proves that Chelation therapy solves the problem of clogging of peripheral circulation in 80% of the cases, the problem of clogging up of the Carotid Artery that prevents blood from reaching the brain, intermittent claudication (leg cramps), and reverses Osteoporosis, placing calcium back into bones and teeth, where they belong.

Osteoporosis often accompanies some form of arthritis. Until early adulthood, more bone is built than is absorbed. But by the mid-30's, both men and women begin to experience a slight and gradual loss of bone mass. After menopause, women lose bone mass much more rapidly — six times more rapidly than men. Then, around age 65, the rate of bone loss slows. One million three hundred thousand women annually suffer from bone fractures due to Osteoporosis. One out of four women are now, or will be victims of this condition. Through the general medical acceptance of Chelation Therapy, such suffering would be totally unnecessary.

In the Cypher, Inc. Chelation Study, 20,000 patients came from many different clinical settings, and they represented patients with a wide diversity of disease conditions.

The cost of the study, funded privately, was high, and not paid by any pharmaceutical company.

The main ingredient, a chemical titled in brief as EDTA (Ethylene Diamine Tetraacetic Acid), is not protected by patent. No pharmaceutical company can pay large returns to stockholders from its sale. No heart surgeon can recover tens of thousands of dollars applying it to heart problems. No hospital can submit bills of tens of thousands of dollars for use of its operating rooms and services, when it is used.

The chemical EDTA, an amino acid, acts like a magnet for positively charged calcium and other metal ions. The chemical EDTA "claws" onto the metallic ions and converts to a chemical that is solvent, safe and easily washed through urine.

A mixture of EDTA and vitamins and minerals is placed in an intravenous solution, and the patient takes an intravenous drip for about 3-1/2 hours as an out-patient. The patient usually sits beside others who may watch television or read or simply visit with one another.

It takes about 20 to 22 treatments for first results to make themselves known to the patient. Depending on severity of the patient's overall problems, he/she may need 30, 40,....., 100 treatments given, usually, at the rate of about three per week.

For the treatment to be maximally effective, good dietary habits and appropriate exercise are important. Alcohol, drugs and smoking will reverse the whole process, again causing free-radical damage that leads to atherosclerosis and subsequent disease problems that occur as a secondary condition of the inability of cells to receive their proper nourishment.

Any drug can be dangerous under the right conditions, to the right person. Even milk can be exceptionally dangerous to one who is allergic to it. According to the manner in which drug safety is determined EDTA is about 3-1/2 times safer or less toxic than taking aspirin. This measure is taken from a standard known as the LD-50, the Lethal Dosage at which 50% of experimental animals will die.

Fifty food companies around the world place EDTA in their canned goods, packaged goods, container liquids, bottles of fruit drinks, baby food and other items for human consumption. EDTA is already an integral part of our daily lives.

As with any other treatment, it can be misused by those who do not follow a proper treatment protocol, and I recommend using the protocol developed by The American College of Advancement in Medicine.

Soap is a chelator, taking off grime and dirt. When you soften water through a house water-softener, you use a chelating agent to take out minerals. EDTA, when used in your 100,000 miles of internal plumbing called capillaries, veins and arteries, acts in a similar manner, by taking out metal ions that will otherwise damage us.

Physical exercise results in production of a natural chelator: lactic acid.

Pollutants we are exposed to over a lifetime from food, air, water and drugs collect in various tissues, in various ways. Tissues from every part of the body are affected, including the brain.

When EDTA chelates out many of these pollutants we find that we can now handle problems better than before and are healthier. Gradually, free radicals affect tissues so that localized accumulations of lipid-containing (fat) material (atheromas) within or beneath the intima (lining of vessels) surfaces of blood vessels clog up the 100,000 miles of capillaries, veins and arteries.

When a fluid flows through a pipe or tube, the rate of flow depends on the diameter of the tube. The smaller the diameter, the faster the flow and the higher the right angle pressure and the lower the internal flow pressure. The rate of flow will increase by a power of three for each unit increase in the diameter, and there will be substantial increase in vascular wall blood pressure. This means that a very, very small decrease in the diameter of the tube increases the flow of the fluid and pressure relatively drastically. Since a smaller vascular opening requires higher blood pressure to flow through, more work is placed on the heart and vascular system. With increased clogging of the circulatory system, therefore, our blood pressure increases.

As atherosclerosis progresses, and the pipes — the capillaries, arteries and veins — decrease in size, each cell of our body also receives considerably less nourishment than before partial clogging, for numerous reasons. There is literally less opportunity to bring molecular food particles to each cell. With less food to each cell, the cell has less capacity to function. Less functioning of each cell means less ability to resist disease and stress, and less ability to repair damage already done. That, of course, means increased opportunity for every kind of disease!

The diseases that chelation can help as a matter of routine include many of the intransigents. Instead of cutting off a gangrenous leg, the leg is healed. Instead of expensive heart bypass surgery, the patient is healed. Instead of Carotid Artery bypass, the brain is again nourished. Senility can be reversed provided brain cells have not been starved of oxygen to the point where they have died. Other diseases that stem from failing organs due to lack of nourishment, including the skin, may be halted or reversed.

There are tens of thousands of good case histories which will not be reported in this book. I refer you to *The Chelation Answer* by Morton Walker, D.P.M. (or one by Walker and Ross). You will be pleased and delighted with its contents and revelations.

The primary reason why I recommend Chelation Therapy to you when you have arthritis has to do with its ability to restore your vital functions. Virtually everyone has some degree of clogging up of the 100,000 miles of plumbing. Often the process of atherosclerosis begins in children's arteries and progresses through adulthood, so that even the finest physical specimens show evidence of this beginning on autopsy. It is virtually certain that you have some of this clogging, to some degree, and that it contributes to your disease at least indirectly.

Anything you can do to better nourish individual cells, you should do, to relieve the burdens that you already carry, and make it easier to fight off the great crippler. But more — EDTA will also help you eliminate many of the pollutant metals that you have acquired over a lifetime and the same that contribute in so many ways to your overall condition, and, by stimulating a gland called the parathyroid, your body will reverse the flow of calcium to harden bones and teeth.

There is another reason why Chelation Therapy is recommended. Whenever we have a flare-up of Rheumatoid Disease, we produce through those inflammatory products a whole host of free-radicals. Free-radicals are actually the damaging agents that attack tissues, such as cartilage. They begin decomposition. That decomposition leads to further secondary free-radicals and that in turn creates further decomposition and tissue sickness. We find ourselves at a point in which the rate at which we can repair damage becomes less than the rate at which the damage is formed — and that results in pain and crippling.

With any severe attack of Rheumatoid Disease, one ought to be able to receive a chelating treatment to minimize free-radical damage.

Chelation therapy will not cure Rheumatoid disease!

It will reduce the damaging products of Rheumatoid Disease temporarily while you develop means for actually halting progress of the disease through our treatment, better nutrition, good health rules and so on.

Chelation therapy will reduce the burden on your organs and glands to help fight the disease. Chelation may solve other medical problems as well as secondary problems related to Rheumatoid Disease.

Before firt trying Chelation Therapy, I prepared a detailed list of symptoms. I also planned to have made periodic laboratory tests during the course of my treatments. I wanted to be able to evaluate for myself what was true or not true about this new form of treatment.

Since I didn't know what the treatment would do, I simply wrote down everything I didn't like about myself or felt was physically or emotionally wrong. I included things on the list which did not change under Chelation therapy. But those symptoms that did change were quite striking and are among symptoms that no amount of traditional drug treatment would have solved.

After having halted the progress of Rheumatoid Arthritis, I was still extremely fatigued. This was a product of the disease, not a product of the medicine I'd taken. I had to lie down at three o' clock every afternoon to rest for three to six hours. I often felt like the world could come to an end, and I'd care less. As an arthritic I'm sure you know the feeling.

I also noted that whenever I lay down to rest, my legs cramped up terribly. The pain and cramping are known as "claudication", and can be a product of calcium insufficiency and/or oxygen lack, both of which can stem from lack of proper cellular nourishment.

I had one joint on one little finger that would not respond to intraneurals or various medicines tried by my family doctor. Probably the reason — deduced after the fact — is that iron from blood leakage acted as a catalyst that cycled through a chemical reaction resulting in the decomposition of the cartilage. It could not be halted without chelating out the iron catalyst.

After three treatments by Chelation Therapy, the little finger joint inflammation disappeared entirely, for the first time in two years. Claudication disappeared at about 22 treatments given over eight weeks. It didn't disappear suddenly, but rather gradually over several treatments, the cramping and pain lessening each time.

Extreme tiredness disappeared after 30 to 40 treatments, ten to fourteen weeks.

I repeat: no other known treatment — no amount of taking of known drugs to control symptoms — could have done the same job.

All improvements have stayed with me, but as a precautionary measure I have taken about 124 treatments. Chelation Therapy, now used on hundreds of thousands, is the medicine of the future, as it is a repair and preventative procedure. If Chelation Therapy, using EDTA, is not used in the future, then one similar to it, or one that performs the same function, will be.

Many of alternative/complementary physicians use Chelation Therapy in their practice.

Chapter XI
Food Allergies

Food allergies contribute to Rheumatoid Disease

symptoms — and may even cause some of the symptoms.

Food allergies are now classified in alternative medicine under the heading of Clinical Ecology, where the environmental causes of allergic symptoms are unraveled.

Certain allergy symptoms have sources that are well known, and easily found, such as those causing "hay fever" which springs from the pollen of ragweed, pigweed, grasses, trees and so on. This is an "external" allergy, as opposed to an "internal" allergy that springs from reactions from substances inside the body. External allergies do not usually cause symptoms of Rheumatoid Arthritis, but they can sure aggravate the condition.

External allergies can be discovered by the detective work of mixing together suspected allergens and after preparing the solution properly, inserting the pollen extract just beneath the skin, where the size and severity of welts determines whether or not an individual is allergic to a particular protein.

Other external sources can be almost anything: gases, fluids, various proteins. Some people develop an allergy to something as common as the gas from a gas stove, and cannot live near or by such sources.

People range from very, very sensitive to not sensitive at all, in a gradient scale. People vary considerably as to what they are allergic to.

The interesting part about allergies is that foods which were perfectly safe for much of our lives suddenly become intolerable — for no obvious reasons.

Early on in the treatment of allergies, professional allergists had great success in testing for and finding common allergens, such as from the pollens of various plants. However, when similar tests were developed for foods, there was, at best, very inconsistent results. Even today I talk with numerous RD victims who tell me that they know they are not allergic to certain foods, because their skin-patch tests did not indicate it. Or, that they are allergic to a certain food, because their skin tests indicate so.

There has been a quiet revolution on the subject of food allergies and testing since 1965 started in part by Theron Randolph, M.D. and four others who organized the Society for Clinical Ecology. By 1980 this society attracted 250 members. Dr. Randolph in part inherited his knowledge and in part created the modern forms of food testing used by Clinical Ecologists. He, more than any other individual, will receive credit for this major contribution to modern medicine.

I've mentioned food allergies to arthritics from time to time, and they often slough it off, as I did at first. There are claims, of course, that solving food allergies will also solve the arthritic processes, halting it. Some of these claims may be absolutely correct — and some may be from a situation where symptoms are merely relieved for secondary reasons.

I think that the relationship between allergies and Rheumatoid Disease is intertangled, and probably operates like this: Like poor nutrition, a food allergy will indeed depress the immunological system with toxins and other chemical burdens such that a borderline arthritic will indeed come down with arthritis on exposure to these additional burdens. After having them lifted, by being relieved of the allergens — by not eating foods to which one is allergic — the arthritic will appear to recover from arthritis, thus it appearing also that the initial cause of the arthritis was the allergy.

I think that in most instances allergens are developed as a secondary condition to having had either Rheumatoid Arthritis or Candidiasis, or both.

According to Paul Reilly, N.D. of Tacoma, WA, "Diet affects bowel flora and Gastro-Intestinal tract permeability. Both of these factors can, in turn, affect the amount of endotoxins (bacterial toxins released from dying bacteria) absorbed. In addition to their . . . role in stimulating B cell mitogenesis, endotoxins are potent activators of the alternate complement pathway, which promotes inflammatory processes. The Kupfer cells of the liver are integral in elimination of circulating immune complexes as well as antigens absorbed intact from the gut. If the liver is not functioning optimally, due to endotoxin damage, these undegraded antigens may be released into the systemic circulation where they can activate further complement release and inflammation." (*Townsend Letter for Doctors and Patients*, Nov. 1986, Issue #42, p.331.)

Allergy reactions also contribute to free-radical pathology, and that extra burden on the body can contribute to arthritic symptoms as well. After all, free-radical pathology, and subsequent damage, is what arthritis is all about. Cleaning up or preventing the development of extra free-radicals, even temporarily, should give some relief, as seems to happen when using EDTA Chelation Therapy, or other means.

If you suspect that you are a candidate for heavy and multiple allergens, from foods and other sources, then you should visit a physician who specializes in Clinical Ecology. The paperback book, *An Alternative Approach to Allergies* by Theron Randolph, M.D. and Ralph W. Moss, Ph.D. is well worth reading.

If you are curious, as I was, as to how much of your Rheumatoid Arthritic pain and reactions stem from food allergies, there is a simple test you can make on yourself that will not require a visit to a physician or to specialists in allergies. Recall that Candidiasis — and probably other causative organisms of Rheumatoid Disease, whatever they might be — both seem to generate food allergies. We know how *Candida albicans* does the job. In the fungus form, it sets roots down into the intestinal mucosa, and thrives there. In doing so, it also opens up minute passages that permit food protein molecules to pass through directly into the bloodstream. In the blood, as a protein molecule, the particle is recognized as an antigen by our defense system. We build antibodies against it, and thus we begin the allergen/antibody warfare — and consequent free-radical generation that affects various tissues adversely.

As time goes on, more protein molecules from different foods enter the blood stream by the same route. The body begins to recognize some different protein molecules as antigens and so it reacts to this food or that food, spreading by a phenomenon known as "cross-reactivity".

Here's how you can find out what foods you are allergic to.

Go on a five day pure water diet. You don't need distilled water, unless you are one of the unfortunate who has a multiplicity of various allergies and must untangle the lot of them extremely accurately. In such a case you need a clinical ecologist, not this simple approach.

I filter my tap-water with a commercial filtration system including activated charcoal and reverse osmosis.

During the five days, every time you get hungry drink more water. Keep filling your stomach with water. The first day will be the hardest, as you will begin to experience withdrawal symptoms from whatever you have been allergic to.

Yes! Allergy reactions are virtually indistinguishable from drug addiction!

At the end of the fifth day, take but one food that you are virtually certain is not an allergen — say, nothing but one species of cold-water fish,

If you have no reaction, then add another food to the fish (or whatever) diet. Continue this process of adding one food each day until you locate one that gives you symptoms of arthritis, headaches, depression, lethargy, diarrhea, or anything else that is unusual.

These symptoms will be caused by the food that is creating your food allergy problem.

You should be cautioned that each trial food must be pure, in the sense that you cannot eat mixtures of any kind. You must read every packaged product to insure that only one ingredient is contained therein. Instead of processed breakfast foods, for example, you must learn to cook, say, just rice, then just oats, then just barley, and so on.

This is a long, detailed process, and it will pay you to take notes.

The reason for the five days, abstinence, is because it takes several days for your body to eliminate every trace of the food that may be creating allergy problems. Any smallest trace will sustain the allergenic symptoms. Then your body needs time to readapt to the non-allergenic state in the absence of the allergen. If five days is more than you can bear, try three days. Anyone can make three full days.

Note taking is a must. Your body could react immediately to an allergen, which is easy to spot. But, it could also react to one that takes three days to kick in. You'll need your log book to find these.

I was purchasing corn on the cob at the supermarket every day. I liked corn, and our treatment protocol for Rheumatoid Arthritis said to eat fresh fruits and vegetables, didn't it?

I was also having diarrhea daily, and had had it for some weeks. This, obviously, was not an allergy, but some other very complex and not well understood medical phenomena. Right?

Wrong!

Had I gone through the traditional medical treatments I probably would have been given some form of feces congealer, or worse. I would never have discovered the answer.

I had typical withdrawal symptoms, and later learned that I was extremely allergic to the corn purchased and eaten almost daily. Every time I ate it, I got diarrhea. So did other corn products create the condition, but not popcorn. You explain it, I can't.

Acorn squash, my mother's favorite, also caused allergic reactions, as did chocolate and oranges. I was not allergic to tangerines or tangelos, however.

When you pass through this test, and no longer eat foods to which you've become allergic, you'll be pleasantly surprised at how much better you feel. You will also relieve your body of a great amount of unnecessary load as you fight your way through solving your Rheumatoid Disease problem.

Many toxins produced from food products and allergens find their way into our system through the lower colon, also. Colonics, which are not in very good repute within establishment medicine, try to scour out these toxins, and yes, people often do feel better after such treatments.

My guess is that the majority of those who seem to need colonics stem from sluggish passage of feces due to improper nutritional intake and/or the use of allergenic foods.

Surprisingly enough, the foods that we like best, those that we purchase time after time, are most likely the foods that we are allergic to. Most chocolateholics — as I tend to be — have a severe allergy to chocolate. Our bodies build up a tolerance, which includes the reconstruction of a physical/chemical state that to some extent resists the allergen. But while doing so, it also builds up a demand that we sense as a desire or wish for the very cause of the state. This is almost a perfect description of drug addiction — and that's what an allergen most represents — a drug addiction. Take away the allergen, and withdrawal symptoms result — as you will learn when you pass through these trials!

The older we get, the more probability of building up various food allergies through commonly used foods. The more allergens we acquire and expose ourselves to, the more free-radical pathology, and the more of that, the more tissue damage, the greater load on our overall systems, the more arthritic — and other — symptoms that weaken us and make us ill.

There are two kinds of food allergy reactions. After several days away from the allergenic food, your body will (1) react immediately with some pain — headache, diarrhea, fever, or something. You'll know you're allergic to it at once. (2) A delayed reaction of several days, perhaps as many as 3. To find these, you must keep a log of foods eaten, and symptoms during the day. Then, by going back and correlating your symptoms with foods consumed several days earlier, one will find the second kind of reaction.

It will pay you, as an arthritic, to take food allergies seriously.

Chapter XII
Bio-detoxification

You should by now feel that one ought to hold no barriers to the search for wellness, but take it where it works and reject it where it does not work, whether found in traditional medicine or not.

The body must maintain wellness functions, such as adequate blood circulation, which is the means to nourish each cell so that cells can properly function. To insure this, we arrived at EDTA Chelation Therapy. The body must rid itself of excessive free-radicals generated via various natural processes. It was built to do so by exercise, as lactic acid formed during exercise is a natural chelator. In the absence of a healthy body with a healthy metabolism, the natural ridding of excess free-radicals seems inherently impossible. To solve that problem also leads to EDTA Chelation Therapy and allergy food challenges as described in prior chapters, as well as good nutritional habits.

Of all the various health processes — nutritional, exercise, medicinal, Chelation Therapy, what have you — none of these can solve the problem of addiction — or the problem of residual poisons accumulated over a life-time that are stored in the fatty parts of our cells.

I learned of the problem of residual toxins stored in fatty parts of cells at a professional medical meeting of the American Academy College for Advancement in Medicine, advocates and researchers of Chelation Therapy.

Whereas EDTA Chelation Therapy solved many hitherto intransigent medical problems, there was a whole class of problems that it would not solve. It seems that residual chemicals that reside in the fatty parts of our cells can come from taking drugs, including medicines, or hard drugs, from the street, or from anesthesia during surgery. Some come from soil and air pollutants, such as found in pesticides and herbicides (remember Agent Orange), consisting of various organic poisons called PCBs, Hexa PCB, PBB, Heptachlor Epoxide, Dieldrin, and so on. Agent Orange is a good example of a chemical that, during its manufacturing processes, collects very small amounts of a dangerous, cancer-forming chemical called Dioxin, that can also create birth defects. This chemical in turn creates for the human effects far beyond its apparent volume and creates the damaging effects for years ahead, perhaps for the individual's lifetime.

Residuals from drugs deliberately taken such as morphine, cocaine, heroin, tobacco and alcohol are also found in the fatty parts of cells.

Consider that the brain consists mainly of fatty (lipids) cells! And that "lipids" are also found every- where throughout the body!

These residual chemicals as stored act as triggers creating large behavior manifestations that simulate every kind of mental, emotional and physical illness.

The very fact that you "like" a particular drug, for example, is an illustration of the triggering action of a chemical that leads you to massive behavioral changes that you would not otherwise make. Try to get tobacco-addicted people off from their cigarette, for example. Listen to their many different and inventive rationalizations.

Or witness the massive behavioral changes that the small residual chemicals create for the tobacco addicted: They stop at the store to buy cigarettes, fumble in purse or wallet for money, carry out the package, start the car, open the package, take out a cigarette and lighter, light the cigarette and inhale deeply blowing smoke out. They put ashes in a tray, and eventually crush the cigarette there, too. This cycle is repeated over and over in some variation — all caused by an illusion called "I want" or "I feel more comfortable with" which is subjectively felt as a desire, and that desire stems from small triggering chemical elements that reside in fatty parts of cells.

I cited the example of tobacco smokers because the addiction is so common, familiar to all, and easily amendable to observation. But all of the other chemicals named, and more, will create similar unconscious behavior manifestations which we are prone to "explain" i.e. rationalize away, after the fact.

By satisfying our subjective "desire" for the chemical involved, our body restores a balance of free-radical pathology that leads to the activation of the consumption in the first instance. This is known as a "homeostasis".

Free-radical pathology, unchecked, leads to extra burdens for arthritics and contributes to their pain and disease. Removing the extra burdens means more bodily systems and organs capable of fighting the great crippler.

When I first heard physicians discussing the shortfalls of using EDTA therapy to solve this particular problem

— as Chelation Therapy "only" solves problems of peripheral circulation and Osteoporosis — I began to pay attention in my readings to possible solutions. Within half a year I learned that L. Ron Hubbard had probably solved the problem back in the late sixties and early seventies under the title of "The Purification Rundown".

I sought for some objective evidence of the results of his invention, which was supplied to me in the form of a published scientific paper entitled "Body Burden Reductions of PCBs, PBBs and Chlorinated Pesticides in Human Subjects" by David W. Schnare, Max Ben and Megan G. Shields in *Ambio*, Vol. 13, No. 5-6, 1984, p. 378.

While I know that scientific jargon is not easy on the eyes or ears for the uninitiated, I think that the scientists' summary of their report is sufficiently revealing to risk its enclosure, which follows:

"With human exposure to environmental contaminants inevitable despite the best application of environmental laws and protection technologies, interest has grown in the potential to reduce the levels of contamination carried in the human host. This study demonstrates the promise of a comprehensive treatment for reduction of body burdens of polychlorinated and polybrominated biphenyls (PCB and PBB) and chlorinated pesticides. Adipose tissue concentrations were determined for seven individuals accidentally exposed to PBB. These patients underwent the detoxification treatment developed by Hubbard to eliminate fat-stored foreign compounds. Of the 16 organohalides examined, 13 were present in lower concentrations at post-treatment sampling. Seven of the 13 reductions were statistically significant; reductions ranged from 3.5 to 47.2 percent, with a mean reduction among the 16 chemicals of 21.3 percent (s.d. 17.1 percent). To determine whether reductions reflected movement to other body compartments or actual burden reduction, a post-treatment follow-up sample was taken four months later. Follow-up analysis showed a reduction in all 16 chemicals averaging 42.4 percent (s.d. 17.1 percent) and ranging from 10.1 to 65.9 percent. Ten of the 16 reductions were statistically significant. Future research stemming from this study should include further investigation of mobilization and excretion of xenobiotics in humans."

In *The California Firefighter* published by the Federated Fire Fighters of California, No. 4, 1984, p. 7, an article titled "Human Detoxification — New Hope for Firefighters" contains information of great interest, because it illustrated how these minute triggering elements, when stored in cellular lipids, can affect our lives grossly.

Those exposed to toxic poisons, such as firefighters, will work normally day to day, when "suddenly" a chronic ailment, disability or disease emerges which, if not fatal, can drastically degrade the quality of living. The Foundation for Advancement in Science and Education (FASE) began studying the toxic bio-accumulation and storage of chemicals in the body and how to reduce the body's burden of stored chemicals. These environmental contaminants can cause perceptual, learning and emotional problems for years following exposure by ingestion, inhaling, through the skin, or other means.

As reported, participants in the FASE study were put through the Hubbard regimen. Upon completion of the program, the Michigan participants revealed significant reductions of all chemicals originally found in their bodies, including PBBs and PCBs. Even more noteworthy were the results of a four- month follow-up examination which demonstrated that the contaminant levels had continued to go down after completion of the program. Dr. David E. Root, an occupational health specialist in Sacramento, CA was Medical Director of the Sacramento Detox Center where many of these tests were conducted.

Of particular interest is the case of Michael Del Puppo, a California police officer who had liquid Phencyclidine (PCP or "angel dust") thrown into his face in the line of duty, a number of years ago. He suffered from severe headaches, memory problems, irritability and fatigue for three years prior to undergoing detoxification at the Los Angeles Detox Center.

For more information on the Hubbard method, check any telephone book in most large cities for The Church of Scientology. Zane Gard, M.D. had to move to Mexico to continue his excellent work, because the local medical board removed his license to practice. They didn't understand the health benefits he was producing by this relatively innocuous therapy. Zane Gard, by the way, has written up numerous case histories of otherwise intransigent cases, many published in *Townsend Letters for Doctors and Patients* but also found at our website. Zane Gard, his wife and daughter were exposed to Agent Orange and sought a method of eliminating the poison and its effects, which led them to Hubbard's method that Dr. Zane Gard then incorporated into a specialty medical practice.

Hubbard's technique is this: Near a sauna he specified about 20 minutes of physical exercise to get blood circulation flowing adequately.Then each participant enters the sauna with temperature between 140 and 180 degrees (F) for about 3-1/2 hours daily for about three to four weeks. Dry sauna is preferred, but you may use a steam or wet sauna if you wish.

The object is to create continuous and copious sweat. It is the sweat elimination system that permits the body to rid itself of deadly toxins stored in the fatty parts of cells.

You are free to leave the sauna anytime, to take a shower, rest in cool air, or to eat lunch — and then return. If you leave simply to escape the heat and sweat, you are cheating yourself, as you'll simply have to endure for a longer number of days until the chore is completed.

The body cannot sweat so long and so copiously without replacing minerals and fluids. Hubbard developed an adjusted vitamin and mineral intake, identifying necessary salts and liquids, including the replacement of "good fats" for the "bad fats" that you wish to sweat out, along with stored toxins.

Before trying this procedure, I'd heard stories of many different and diverse strange phenomena. I'd heard that one experienced (or re-experienced) anesthesia, sunburns (showing up exactly as seen on the beach, swim suit straps and all), hallucinatory images and sensations, and so on. These are what Hubbard called "restimulations of past experiences" from when the drug, radiation or environ-mental pollution was first encountered.

At first I found it extremely difficult to force myself through the rigorous sweat ordeal, and especially the heat, wanting to give myself every excuse — rationalization — for not being there. I would "dope off" in a deep lethargy. Then, as the days passed and I found it easier to exist in the hot-box, I found different sensations occurring. One day I tasted and smelled and had every sensation of again being drugged with nitrogen oxide — laughing gas — which stemmed from only one place. I'd had teeth pulled in a dentist's chair in the nineteen forties.

Another time I re-experienced the sickening smell of ether, this from adenoid surgery in the doctor's office in the nineteen thirties.

Most difficult to explain was another experience, after my day of sweating and about two weeks into the detoxification. I was home, lying on the bed watching television and I perceived that my body, longitudinally through my forehead, nose, chest and crotch, was split by two temperatures. My left side was extremely hot to touch, and the right side quite normal. I'd had two operations on the left side, but I know not why the relationship in splitting the body so neatly. This lasted three hours. Years later it occurred to me that the lymph system is split like this, and the operations on one side somehow related to the lymph system on that side and created the left side fever.

Apparently in a way that I do not yet understand, radiation of various kinds is also stored in these lipids, as witness the phenomena of old sunburn's reappearing.

Hubbard discovered that on completion of the sauna experience, most physical addictions disappeared, leaving only the psychic component that led to the addiction in the first place. This component he proposed to handle by the technology administered by the church, which is another subject in itself.

The essential difference between Hubbard's program and those of medical centers, where the program has been slow in being accepted, is that the medical centers provide periodic laboratory tests to ascertain the current levels of toxins in the lipids. Since there are nearly an infinite number of possible toxins, one must be choosy about what is tested for, or the costs can be excessive.

Hubbard's program relies more on experience coupled with your own intuition, as to when you are through. You can plan, however, on a minimum of about three and one half weeks which can often be scheduled at your convenience, like after working hours.

I can't promise that you will obtain any observable benefits from this program, as I cannot know if you have stored environmental toxins, or that you will release them successfully. However, if you do have such poisons affecting your various systems, and if you do release them successfully, you will surely be better able to fight off Arthritis, or any other disease, for that matter.

Chapter XIII
Stress Management

No subject is more important to wellness than stress management. It is also the subject that physicians ignore, and patients avoid.

Physicians ignore stress management because (1) they are not taught the skills required, (2) it may be exceedingly time consuming, and therefore cut down on patient load, and subsequent income, (3) there are few reliable methods for insuring relief of stress management on every patient, (4) the patient will most likely ignore the advice anyway.

Patients ignore stress management advice because (1) they "know" their problem is physically based, and all they need is a magic pill to achieve wellness, (2) they cannot follow the advice in any case, because their responsibilities, or ethics, or religion, or children, or whatever, require them to hold onto their present employment, their line of work, their husband/wife, their house, et. al. (3) stress management may require confronting one's own emotions, a most deceitfully painful process that will drive a man/woman to lie, steal, cheat, kill, rape and pillage before so facing.

Harsh words! Indeed they are!

There are few physicians living today who will take the time and effort to explore all of the causative relationships in Arthritis. It would take a partnership between the patient and physician such that one would study hormonal imbalances, nutritional problems, allergens, possible infectious agents, stress management,mercury poisoning, root canal infections, and perhaps many other factors unique to that individual.

Such a physician might indeed starve to death, unless the patient is prepared to devote major energies and finances to the task. With your full cooperation, the cost and time can be reduced immensely, and the physician can perform as a coordinator and safety check for those things you wish to try and to learn about yourself.

Many alternative/complementary physicians are holistic minded, and are quite aware of the place that stress plays in diseases, including arthritis. But what do they say to a female patient with the responsibility of raising five children that must be fed daily, clothes cleaned, house prepared, lessons readied, driven to the doctor, and so on?

Or what does one tell the husband who must daily submit himself to a suppressive personality that delights in destroying everything human or creative, a husband who must, nonetheless bring home the bacon for the sake of a demanding wife and five lovely children?

Consider this: In a small family of two children, mother and father, there are 2 raised to the 4th power number of possible interactions, taken just two at a time, or 32 in all. When taken three at a time, there is a total of 37 possible emotional entanglements. Multiply those powers by additional powers of two when counting school teachers, principals, supervisors, friends and non-friends, neighbors and so on, and we humans have tremendously complex social interactions.

Probably the most persistent stress, however, comes directly from work or home, and those are regions where the physician dare not tread — and seldom, too, is the preacher or priest or rabbi permitted to enter there!

Who can leave home or work conveniently, simply to avoid stress?

But stress management, stress elimination, is absolutely essential if we are to get well and stay well as arthritis sufferers. The reason is this: When we are under stress, adrenalin is produced which turns on cortisone in the form of a substance called "cortisol". Cortisol, to provide us with quick energy during emergencies, causes small proteins in the immunological system to be utilized as a quick energy source. When we are under stress continuously, this process goes on continuously. The utlization of portions of the immunological system as quick energy causes the natural balances of cells responsible for defending us from invaders to be upset, and that, in effect, creates a kind of weakening of the immunological system. The weakening of the immunological system permits organisms of opportunity to spread throughout the body, such as the presumed causative organism of Rheumatoid Diseases, *Candida albicans* and so on.

We have already seen how such organisms of opportunity will, in their turn, create their own kinds of havoc, leading to symptoms similar to Arthritis, and to different symptoms and to allergies, and so on.

Reflect seriously on this vicious cycle that is like a snake that feeds on itself. It is a modern wonder that holistic physicians do not concentrate chiefly on stress aspects over the long run!

Some physicians do recognize this important aspect, and they look for a quick and easy fix in the forms of hypnosis, bio-feedback, positive suggestion, support groups for their patients, and so on.

Support groups, I believe, have their place and one day But I doubt that any system of psychotherapy or hypnosis or positive suggestion, or the various "faith" schools, mysticism or self-help regime is useful; and, I believe, sometimes they may be dangerous.

Actually solving the basic problems of stress management requires not so much the changing of the environment surrounding the patient as it does getting the patient to change his/her own inner world. To do this, as I believe Jesus Christ and other great religious pioneers learned, requires a system of techniques for self-confrontation.

These are my opinions, of course, and each one must decide for him/her self. For what it is worth, I find the practice of psychiatry medieval, one that marches to unacceptable standards of workability; I find psychology fragmented and dedicated to means of external controls, as opposed to development of self-respect and self-determinism; hypnosis abhorrent, as it is a technique which, at best, shifts one problem to another sometimes of greater magnitude, and at worst eliminates the essential elements of self- determinism and self-respect. Bio-feed back mechanisms, for the most part, lack cohesiveness and the sense to know what is important and what is not, and further often does not address the patient's source problems, manipulating symptoms rather than causes. I qualify this latter, in that sometimes, under very stringent conditions, bio-feedback might be useful, for limited reasons.

Identifying the symptom with the cause is sort of like magic. It presumes that an identity relationship exists between cause and effect. If the symptom is the symbol of the thing itself, the cause, then by manipulating the symbol of the cause, one proceeds with wellness as the cause can be assumed to be also manipulated successfully whenever the symptom is manipulated successfully.

That is about as much nonsense as arguing that by suppressing the nasal drainage of a cold, the cold is cured!

Let me hasten to add that I am not at all opposed to anything that you, the patient, find worthwhile for eliminating stress from your life and restoring to it meaning and peace of mind. If it works for you, I am most happy, as that is my goal and the goal of the Foundation, to see that you and everyone else in the world who is arthritic get well.

If you find that a particular religious belief and practice does the trick, then by all means enjoy yourself in it. It is exactly what you should do and what you need to do, if it works. If other forms of stress management work, including that of stress clinics, by all means attend them and use them successfully. If you believe that a particular brand of mystic belief or practice of Kung Fu, or Karate or even our chief competitor, the Arthritis Foundation, provides you with the services and help that you need for stress management, then be my guest. Go to it! Get yourself well!

But let's not lie to ourselves that a particular physician, health helper, belief system or hypnotist or anything or anyone is in fact helping us when it or they are not!

There is a pragmatic engineering approach to the art of getting well that relies on specialists, books, articles, insight, but not upon Authority, for Authority demands suspension of self, and blind acceptance of only that which may or may not be true for you.

Many physicians keep a patient returning by means of the physician's overwhelming personality, not results. I can remember one talk I gave on a "talk-back" show on a Chicago radio station with a wide audience. I started to explain the benefits of our treatment protocol and the difficulties when combined with damaging gold treatments.

A very irate lady called who insisted that she'd been to a local rheumatologist and had had gold shots, and declared that I was completely wrong. He was, after all, such a nice doctor and he knew what he was doing.

She could not understand that "niceness" and "Authoritarianism" were not getting her well, and that her blinding mis-placed loyalties were keeping her sick.

Why should she have found it necessary to invest so much emotion and faith and energy in Authority, rather than invest that same emotion and faith and energy in herself?

You may or may not wish to try some of the treatments I recommend in this book. That doesn't matter to me. What matters is that you get the idea that out there, in the real world, are literally thousands of safe and perhaps effective treatments that are being overlooked by our present medical establishment, for whatever reasons. Some of these treatments will be designed exactly for you. You cannot find such treatments without searching for them, and that search must rely on your own self-honesty, to know when it is working and when it is not.

You already know that you will not get well from conventional treatment. Those who treat you say so, as does the Arthritis Foundation. You <u>may</u> not get well with the unconventional. <u>You absolutely will not get well with conventional treatments.</u>

Having stated all of the above, I now return to the very important subject of stress management.

You can make out a list of all of the normal activities and relationships in your daily living that create emotional distress or fatigue. You can attempt to devise ways and means of relieving these yourself.

Sometimes, of course, we are so pressed down by pain, sickness and overwhelming problems that it is impractical to expect us to do this rationally for ourselves, in which case we need a person who is truly interested in our welfare and one who can be relied upon to correctly identify our stress agents, and one who will give appropriate advice on how to change, reduce, or eliminate them.

Social workers, of course, can often help with this approach.

Other social agencies, religious organizations, educators and non-profit foundations may also provide the external advice and assistance that you need.

Others have undertaken the approach of identifying causes of stress — indeed, there are tons of books on the subject to be found at any bookstore or library. I shan't attempt it further.

While some advice that you receive from such sources

may seem painful, or sometimes impossible, to follow, it will nonetheless be painless compared to that of self-confrontation through systematic introspection. Yet, this last approach is in the final analysis what is needed for permanency in our wellness.

Arthritics need rest. Pain and subsequent free-radical pathology resulting from inflammation and pain requires much more rest than is normal. Pick a time of the day when you are the lowest ebb — and you'll know what that means — and lie down to read, listen to the radio, watch and listen to television, or simply sleep. Push every thought from your mind except the need to rest, the need to serve yourself and no one else. You may surprise yourself that this time period does not always require a long time, sometimes but fifteen minutes or so. You'll likely spring up again refreshed and ready to battle the world's tigers.

Also find something that you really enjoy doing, preferably something that provides you with light exercise, or, if you are physically capable of it, heavy exercise.

Exercise is important, and also covered very well in hundreds of other books and booklets. The reason why it's important is that your body needs to increase it's metabolism, and that comes about only through exercise performed daily. A fifteen minute brisk walk can keep your heart-lung systems in grand shape, and help to flush out many toxins that will otherwise bury you.

I used to dance perhaps seven nights per week, usually with the younger set. I was 63 (1988) and I did country and western style, John Travolta-type disco, ballroom, swing, jitterbug, bop, you name it. When I could find the time I was learning to tap-dance, and even if a bad tap dancer I could learn a soft-shoe-shuffle!

This Foundation's viewpoint is that exercise is not appropriate unless you've halted the progress of Rheumatoid Disease, as vigorous exercise seems to spread the disease faster, what is known as "galloping" arthritis.

After your disease is halted, exercise daily in whatever manner is safe for you, and that you find pleasant.

Exercise, itself, is a kind of stress management.

You may not like dancing, or may be crippled so that you cannot do this kind of exercise. Don't feel sorry for yourself, as that simply adds to stress burdens. There is almost always some form of exercise that you can do: walking, hobbling, running, bodily exercises in or out of water, Jaccusi, bicycling, swimming, ballgames, pushups with either feet or hands or both, barbells while sitting in a wheelchair. Unless you are completely paralyzed there will be something that you can do that is beneficial, and will get the heart and lungs in shape and keep it that way. If it is also pleasant, you've found another plus, for there is nothing worse than an exercise done for its own sake.

The second and possibly most important approach to stress management lies with your inner world, which is the last unexplored frontier, one inch behind the skull.

You and I got the way we are because of what we are (genetics) and what was done to us (environment).

But we also got the way we are because of what we have decided for ourselves. If this paradox disturbs you, then you, like me, have much to learn!

We are all self-determined. Self-determination means more than simply getting our own way, which is selfishness. Self-determination means that everything in life that has happened to us must be viewed from an inner world as though we brought it on ourselves — rather than rationalize away the responsibilities inherent in our choice and lot, we should strive to see how it might be that we are responsible for our present state.

We arthritics, like everyone else, do not want to admit our shortcomings that create stress through our own decisions and actions. We may not want to admit it, but our personalities leave much to be desired. We are angry people, capable of destructive action. We dwell in the past, rather than the present or future. We express hate and we strive to suppress pain, to hold onto all the motion that might be around us or within us, to stop pain. We often disagree with others' views of reality, hastening to disagree before we've considered all factors. If we fail to destroy others' or others' view of reality, we often turn on ourselves, or on our environment. Even when our intentions are stated to be good, we often bring about destruction, but we'll blame others or the situation or the environment for our prior decisions and failures. We often lie, not just to others, but to ourselves, and we'll often assume responsibility to destroy. We'll begin a task strongly, but weaken quickly, we accept alarming remarks literally and have a brutal sense of humor. We often use threats, punishments and alarming lies to dominate others. We negate against others' remarks, but absorb them. We seldom experience any pleasures.

You will agree with me that the above list of characteristics for arthritics is not a very favorable image, but anyone who suffers from eternal pain, as we do, will have some of those characteristics. What is involved are things that have been done to us, not that we wish to be the way we are. It takes a great deal of effort — energy and attention — to control these "negative" characteristics so that we place a "proper face" on our social behavior.

That necessity to control our worse impulses also places us under more stress!

Perhaps you will find this facet of getting well the most difficult, but we must take responsibility for our attitudes, emotions, sicknesses, and every aspect of our living.

We must decide whether or not we wish to survive! — and all else follows accordingly.

Chapter XIV
Sclerotherapy (Proliferative) Therapy

While intraneural injections are the treatment of choice in the Foundation's protocol for the pain of Rheumatoid Disease and Osteoarthritis, they do not always halt the pain permanently for a variety of reasons, among which is the fact that basic causes of the nerve lesions may not yet be solved.

Two of our former referral physicians, Harold C. Walmer, D.O. (Elizabethtown, PA) and W.W. Mittlestadt, M.D., D.O. (Ft. Lauderdale, FL) brought to my attention another source of pain and problems not often recognized — and a possible solution for them.

Later another physician, William J. Faber, D.O. mailed to the Foundation interesting literature related to a book he is writing on the subject. If, after reading this section, you have further interest in his forthcoming publication. You can order his and Morton Walker's book.

There is often much damage to ligatures, tendons, muscles, joints and joint cartilage during episodes of Rheumatoid Disease and also throughout Osteoarthritis. Much of this damage has hitherto been unresolvable.

It is possible, but not probable, that an arthritic will

also suffer from Gout or what is often known as "Gouty Arthritis".

Those who have gouty arthritis have an inability to excrete as much uric acid crystals as they should through their urine. These almost undissolvable crystals precipitate out in joints, and create extreme pain each time one moves, like sharp, small needles lodged therein. One of our recmmended medicines, Allopurinol, is traditionally used to prevent the formation of these crystals. Another, the trademarked ColBENEMID, containing a mixture of Probenecid and Colchicine, helps the body to eliminate the crystals. A combination of the two will halt the precipitation of the uric acid crystals, and also help to rid the body of the painful crystals. Gout seems to be caused by infection of mycoplasmal bacteria which produces ubiquiton, a substance that causes excessive precipitation of uric acid crystals.

As an incidental, one of the drugs in ColBENEMID was serendipitously discovered to help the liver to heal. You will read more about Colchicine in a later chapter.

One set of joint pains that disturbs some of us greatly cannot be attributed any longer to active Rheumatoid Disease or Gout. Usually this pain is the result of having had either Rheumatoid Disease or Osteoarthritis, and stems from the absence of cartilage, the friction of bone on bone (clicking joints as we move them), weakened tendons, ligatures and muscles where they should attach to bone surfaces through tearing, stretching or physical damage.

Dr. Faber explains: "X-rays cannot show anything but bones, and do not show torn ligaments which stabilize joints by holding bones in place. When ligaments are torn they are unable to effectively function to hold bones in place which causes friction as bone rubs against bone.

"The body attempts to correct this problem caused by the torn ligaments by creating 'arthritis'. In this instance 'arthritis' — (including pain from calcium spurs: Ed.) — is the body's attempt to compensate for the torn ligament's inability to hold the bones in place.

"This," says Faber, "explains why anti-inflammatory drugs and cortisone are often not effective. Excess friction, not inflammation, is the cause of the joint pain. Reducing inflammation will not eliminate the problem nor provide long-term relief. Only strengthening the ligaments will correct the problem."

Since ligaments contain no muscle fibers, exercise also will not correct the problem or provide long-term relief.

When should "proliferative" therapy be considered? According to Faber, under the following conditions.

1. When ligaments are either lax or torn, then the ligaments can be strengthened.

2. When any joint has pain lasting longer than six weeks. A healthy body should be able to heal torn or lax ligaments within six weeks. If joint pain persists beyond six weeks, it is an indication that the body has not been able to handle it on its own and that the joint is unstable from lax or torn ligaments.

3. Any joint that is helped by a support or brace. A brace or support functions as ligaments do. That is, they function to stabilize the joint. If a support brace helps, proliferative therapy is indicated as it strengthens the ligaments, enabling the necessary support.

4. Any joint that fails to respond to manipulation or adjustments. Many joint problems can be resolved with

manipulation/adjustments and often manipulation/ adjustment is the treatment of choice. Manipulation is highly effective when bones are out of alignment as a result of bad posture or injury. When manipulation or adjustment doesn't provide lasting relief it is because the ligaments are lax or torn and can't hold the joint in place.

5. Any joint that is worse after surgery. When injured joint spacers are removed in surgery (discs, cartilage) this causes the ligaments to become lax. This laxity causes the joint to become unstable and eventually form arthritis.

6. Any joint that is better with rest and worse with exercise. Rest allows the body to heal itself and also reduces friction which is caused by a torn or lax ligament in a weakened joint. Exercise of an unstable joint makes it hurt more as it creates increased friction. Because of the decreased blood supply in ligaments, rest alone is often not sufficient for the body to heal itself. And, because ligaments and tendons do not contain muscle fiber, exercise will not heal an injured ligament or tendon.

7. Any popping, snapping or clicking joint. A joint that is unstable snaps, clicks or pops. Proliferative therapy causes strengthening of the ligaments and thus stabilizes the joint thus eliminating the popping, snapping and/or clicking.

8. Any torn tendon or tendonitis that does not resolve after six weeks. Tendons are like ligaments in that they are fibrous tissue and they attach to the bone. They also have a lack of blood supply like ligaments, and therefore have a poor healing ability. Proliferative therapy causes a permanent strengthening of torn or lax tendons just as it does for torn or lax ligaments.

In this form of treatment, medical specialists (M.D., D.O.) often utilize x-ray, photographs and thermography (infra-red mapping of body inflammation through heat sources). Such practitioners become very skilled at locating hot spots (inflammation and pain) by sense of touch, to confirm results of other tests.

After locating all the body points that require this form of treatment, a fine needle that does not convey a great deal of pain is used to insert close to the bursar sacs — at the joints at the junction of bones and ligaments — a combination mixture of procaine and sodium morrhuate.

The procaine acts as an immediate pain desensitizer (as it also does in intra-neural therapy) and the body eventually converts it to a Vitamin B which is then easily utilized to good purpose. The sodium morrhuate is a natural body substance which the body uses to promote the growth of fibroblasts and collagen tissue, both necessary to reattach and/or strengthen tendons and ligaments to the bone. Fibro-blasts are cells or tissues from which connective tissue is grown. Collagen is a fibrous insoluble protein found in connective tissue, including skin, bone, ligaments and cartilage, and represents about 30% of the total body protein.

Whether or not these substances do as described is no longer under scientific question, as the University of Iowa, and other locations, conducted tests on animals presumably not subject to human placebo effects, and the treatment worked on them, promoting the growth of fibroblasts and collagen tissue at the sites of injection.

The treatment is taught only in post-doctoral courses, however, and it is unlikely that the average family physician would know its benefits, or how to perform the tasks.

With some patients there have been remarkable improvements after but a single treatment, unless the individual does not have good healing abilities (poor metabolism) in which case many of the Foundation's foregoing treatments (and perhaps others) should be considered respecting nutrition and other good health habits.

It usually takes 6 to 12 sessions to fully strengthen a small joint in most cases. While relief may come early, correction comes only after the joint is fully strengthened. Large joints such as the hip or back usually require 12 to 24 sessions for correction. The elbow and wrist about 12 to 24 sessions as these are high stress areas. Treatment times vary and may take longer if the patient previously received cortisone or in case of severe injury or re-injury. Each session increases strength.

The therapy is safe, natural and effective in experienced hands. Lessening of pain should result as well as strengthening of joints.

The treatment should be considered as an adjunct to other treatments for Osteoarthritis, compression fractures, rotator cuff tears, unstable knees, backs, neck, shoulders, hips, wrists and elbows that have been operated on unsuccessfully, and certainly if possible, to do before operations are even considered.

I have had a great deal of joint damage in shoulders and spine, and so naturally I was interested in Faber's, Mittlestadt's and Walmer's recommendations that I attend a man skilled in this therapy nearby.

I was referred to J.A. Carlson, D.O., of Knoxville, TN, (deceased) who specialized in non-surgical orthopedics using the above described therapy and others for the practice of Musculo-Skeletal and Athletic Medicine.

I should mention that former Surgeon General Koop

used this treatment to heal his back.

Chapter XV
Vitamin C — the Great Missing Vitamin

One of the great anti-oxidants is Vitamin C, and deserves its own special chapter.

Everyone is probably familiar with Linus Pauling's book, *Vitamin C and the Common Cold* published by W.H. Freeman and Company and available through virtually all book stores in paperback.

Much original work with large dosages of Vitamin C was done by Fred R. Klenner, M.D. of Reidsville, NC. Dr. Klenner found that viral diseases could be cured by intravenous sodium ascorbate in amounts up to 200 grams per 24 hours. Irwin Stone (*The Healing Factor*) pointed out the significance of Vitamin C in the treatment of many diseases, and also that humans were unable to synthesize ascorbate, resulting in the medical condition called hypoascorbemia — diseases attributed to or caused by the insufficiency of Vitamin C. Linus Pauling, Ph.D., reviewed the literature on Vitamin C and led the crusade to make it known to the public and the medical profession. Ewing Cameron in association with Linus Pauling showed the usefulness of ascorbate when treating cancer. (*Cancer and Vitamin C*)

It is of great significance that humans, primates, guinea pigs and a very small number of bird species are unable to synthesize Vitamin C. An easy conclusion to reach is that all of these mammals passed through an evolutionary period where each lost the ability to synthesize Vitamin C.

Irwin Stone described the genetic defect whereby higher primates lost the ability to synthesize ascorbate as caused by a mutated defective gene for the liver enzyme L-gulonolactone oxidase. All higher mammals except primates, guinea pigs and the few bird species mentioned developed a bio-chemical feedback mechanism which causes an increase in ascorbate synthesis under the influence of external or internal stresses.

One of our former referral physicians, Robert F. Cathcart, M.D., in his paper "Vitamin C, Titrating to Bowel Tolerance, Anascorbemia, and Acute Induced Scurvy", *Medical Hypotheses* 7:1359-1376, 1981, presents his brilliantly developed clinical findings that demonstrated rather clearly how the body tolerates increasing amounts of Vitamin C when under the stress of various diseases. He shows from his clinical findings on 9,000 patients that the body's ability to absorb Vitamin C is directly proportional to the severity of stress and/or disease. Diseases improve or are cured by his "bowel tolerance" measuring technique for determining the exact amount of Vitamin C required by the body at the moment, and he will label a "100 gram cold", for example, when the cold requires 100 grams to be rid of its symptoms, a "50 gram cold" when it takes but 50 grams, and so on.

Mammals that do not have the ability to synthesize Vitamin C are at a distinct disadvantage, and obviously can be affected by external organisms and stress more easily than those that can synthesize their Vitamin C. Those that do so, synthesize Vitamin C with a precision that would shame most scientific laboratories.

They manufacture and meter out throughout their bodily systems exact quantities of Vitamin C dependent upon their present degree of stress and their degree of need for a given set of infections.

The more infection and/or stress, the more Vitamin C is manufactured. The less infection and/or stress, the less Vitamin C is manufactured.

Have you ever wondered how it is that certain pets, like dogs and cats, can literally eat bacteria-ridden garbage and, providing they are not poisoned, they have no difficulty in staying healthy?

Whether establishment physicians accept the fact or not, tens of thousands — no hundreds of thousands — have already verified good results through usage of Vitamin C. Many of our referral physicians know and use these techniques to fight infection, reduce stress and to assist the immunological system.

When using EDTA Chelation Therapy, Vitamin C along with other vitamins and minerals are added. Vitamin C can be used intravenously by itself in sufficiently large dosages to reverse a number of otherwise intransigent disorders that have a causation based on free-radical pathology.

Cathcart says: "Well nourished humans contain not much more than 5 grams of Vitamin C in their bodies. The majority of people have much less, and therefore are at risk for many problems related to failure of metabolic processes that depend on ascorbate. Stone calls this condition 'chronic subclinical scurvy'.

"Some of the increased need for ascorbate," Cathcart relates, "occurs in areas of the body not primarily involved in the disease and can be accounted for by such functions as the adrenals producing more adrenalin and corticoids; the immune system producing more antibodies, interferon, and other substances to fight infection; the macrophages utilizing more ascorbate with their increased activity; and production and protection of a substance called c-AMP and c-GMP with subsequent increased activity of other endocrine glands, and so on." Cathcart continues with ". . . there must be a tremendous draw on ascorbate locally by increased metabolic rates in the primarily infected tissues. The infecting organisms themselves liberate toxins which are neutralized by ascorbate, but in the process destroy ascorbate. The levels of ascorbate in the nose, throat, eustachian tubes and bronchial tubes locally infected by a 100 gram cold must be very low, indeed. With this acute induced scurvy localized in these areas, it is small wonder that healing can be delayed and complications such as chronic sinusitis, otitis media and bronchitis, etc. develop."

Cathcart adds that from his personal experience and from that of patients, it is apparent that the adrenals are capable of utilizing large amounts of ascorbate with benefit if made available.

According to Cathcart, the following medical problems should be expected with increased incidence as ascorbate is depleted: "disorders of the immune system such as secondary infections, Rheumatoid Arthritis and other collagen disease, allergic reactions to drugs, foods and other substances, chronic infections such as herpes, or sequelae of acute infections such as Guillain-Barre' and Reye's syndromes, rheumatic fever, or scarlet fever; disorders of the blood coagulation mechanisms such as hemorrhage, heart attacks, strokes, hemorrhoids, and other vascular thrombosis; failure to cope properly with stresses due to suppression of the adrenal functions such as phlebitis, other inflammatory disorders, asthma and other allergies; problems of disordered collagen formation such as impaired ability to heal, excessive scarring, bed sores, varicose veins, hernias, stretch marks, wrinkles, perhaps even wear of cartilage or degeneration of spinal discs; impaired function of the nervous system such as malaise, decreased pain tolerance, tendency to muscle spasms, even psychiatric disorders and senility; and cancer from the suppressed immune system and carcinogens not detoxified; etc."

Sounds like all of the good features of a popular patent medicine at the old-tyme-medicine-show, doesn't it?

Cathcart does not say that ascorbate depletion was the only cause for the diseases above, but that a lack of the Vitamin can predispose to these diseases and that each one of the systems involved in the above diseases are known to be dependent upon ascorbate to function properly. Further, that patient improvement has been noted when Vitamin C has been provided in proper amounts by himself and others, including A. Kalokerinos and F.R. Klenner (*Every Second Child*).

All readers should rush out to the local health food store and purchase Vitamin C tablets. Right? Wrong!

The problem with tablets is this: Tablets contain ascorbic acid or Sodium or Calcium ascorbate crystals held together by binders. If you were to take a sufficient amount of ascorbic acid in this form to alleviate most conditions, you would discover yourself with diarrhea from the binders alone, and this would happen long before you determined the correct dosage of Vitamin C for your present condition.

Vitamin C is also often quite expensive when purchased in tablet form from local health food outlets. You need to find a source of ascorbate that is reasonably low cost, without binders, and purchase it in large quantities, so that you feel free to add the Vitamin C to your diet as a supplement each day. How much you should take is to be determined by your physical condition, amount of stress, whether or not seriously ill, and so on. The means of determining this amount will be described via Cathcart's "Bowel Titration" technique.

Another fact you should know is that ascorbic acid, sodium ascorbate and calcium ascorbate are physiologically equivalent with ascorbic acid being, weight for weight, slightly more concentrated.

One good source for all three of the above is from Bronson Parmaceuticals. You can order soluble, fine crystals of Vitamin C in 1 kilo quantities for ascorbic acid and sodium ascorbate, and in 1 pound quantity for calcium ascorbate.

You will find it to your advantage to have all three, as the ascorbic acid can be added to fruit drinks and other fluids where the sodium and calcium ascorbate would not taste quite right, and vice versa. The two ascorbates are virtually tasteless (with a very light salty flavor, if anything), and the ascorbic acid is tart, as an acid should be.

All three can be mixed in water.

To avoid overbalancing mineral ratios, by taking too much sodium as compared to calcium, one can mix the two ascorbates, sodium and calcium — and one can also supplement with magnesium and whatever minerals that your physician recommends, the magnesium in dosages of 1/2 by weight of the calcium intake.

Cathcart's "Bowel Tolerance" technique is simple to apply. A normal person can probably get by very well on between 4 and 15 grams per 24 hour period. This includes, of course, the amounts you consume via green peppers, lettuce, fruits and so on.

When one comes down with a sickness, or has been under unusual stress, one increases the amount of Vitamin C consumed within 24 hours to the point where diarrhea just begins — then one backs off to the dosage used just prior to the diarrhea. That "just lower than" is the exact amount your body needs for the time being.

It may be necessary to increase your dosages by amounts of 5, 10, 15, . . . grams per 24 hour period until you find the correct dosage. These are monitoring matters best left up to you and your personal experiences.

I usually take 1 gram in the morning, afternoon and evening or between 3 and 5 grams per day, as a regular maintenance routine. It is easy and convenient — using a 1/4 measuring teaspoon laying beside one of the Vitamin C containers — to quickly slip 1 gram into my ice-water.

You can add the same quantity, or more, to a glass of orange juice, or any other fruit juices, but I would recommend using ascorbic acid, as it is the natural taste of fruits.

As presented at the Second Annual Rheumatoid Disease Foundation Medical Seminar, Cathcart's findings were:

	Usual Bowel Tolerance Doses	
Condition	Grams Per 24 Hours	Number of Doses Per 24 Hours
Normal	4-15	4
Mild Cold	30-60	6-10
Severe Cold	60-100	8-15
Influenza	100-150	8-20
ECHO, Coxsackievirus	100-150	8-20

Mononucleosis	150-200+	15-25
Viral Pneumonia	100-200+	15-25
Hay Fever, Asthma and Food Allergy	0.5-50	4-8
Burn, Injury, Surgery	25-150	6-20
Anxiety, Exercise and Other Mild Stresses	15-25	4-6
Cancer	15-100	4-15
Ankylosing Spondylitis	15-100	4-15
Reiter's Syndrome	15-60	4-10
Acute Anterior Uveitis	30-100	4-15
Rheumatoid Arthritis	15-100	4-15
Bacterial Infections	30-200+	10-25
Infectious Hepatitis	30-100	6-15
Candida Infections	15-200+	6-25

According to Cathcart, disease symptoms will persist until the amount of Vitamin C reaches about 80-90% of bowel tolerance dosages. Perhaps it is only near this tolerance that the ascorbate is pushed into the primary sites of the disease.

Further, suppression of symptoms in some instances may not be total, but usually it is very significant and often the amelioration is complete and rapid.

If you try this procedure and find that your bowels emit a great deal of gas to the point of discomfort as you increase daily dosages, then you are one who has "gas-forming" microflora throughout your intestines, such as, but not only as, *Candida albicans*. The gas is carbon dioxide, usually, a by-product of yeast organisms, and others. This indicates a problem that should be handled if you are to have good absorption of digested foods, and if you are to successfully use the Cathcart technique.

According to Cathcart, the Bowel Tolerance test should be made only with ascorbic acid, but once the tolerance dosage is learned, for that particular problem, then you can use the other ascorbates. For general maintenance dosages, either ascorbic acid or the sodium or calcium ascorbates are O.K.

As I've mentioned earlier, every person responds to substances differently, and Vitamin C is no exception. According to Cathcart, at least 80% of his patients tolerated ascorbic acid well. Perhaps among those who did not are those who also had the gas generation problem from organisms that did not belong to the human symbiote family.

Evidently Vitamin C when taken properly can provide an important supplement to restoring the body's natural health just as EDTA Chelation Therapy restores the ability of the cell to nourish itself.

While degenerative arthritis will sometimes be improved, it is the various inflammatory Rheumatoid Diseases where most improvement shows. There are probably several reasons why. There is first the general free-radical scavenging effect of Vitamin C that can temporarily at least clean-out inflammatory products and toxins. Then there is the fact that Vitamin C when placed in all organs and tissues in appropriate amounts for a given person will permit the bodily functions to behave properly. Third, there is the fact of eliminating altogether, or at least reducing attacks on, tissues by foreign invaders, thus helping ourselves in the restoration of health or to maintain health. There is also a related factor, where Vitamin C can block allergic reactions with augmented adrenal functions, and allergic reactions may be prevalent in a large number of Rheumatoid Arthritis patients as well as Candidiasis patients. Finally, and maybe most important, the ability to relieve stress that produces continuous and damaging cortisol via the adrenal glands.

Maintenance dosages are difficult for a physician to state properly, as the individual needs of the patient vary so, and further the needs vary considerably in terms of degree of stress and sickness. Each Rheumatoid Arthritis victim must learn and make dosage determination for self.

One last point, from personal experience: I once poo-poohed use of large quantities of Vitamin C as I was taught by very well meaning "establishment" physicians that I got sufficient vitamins and minerals in my daily foods.

I didn't question at the time how others could know this when they did not follow me about daily to see how badly I ate.

I took Vitamin C in tablet form only a few milligrams per day, and saw absolutely no effect on colds. Not until reading Cathcart, Pauling, Stone and others did I realize how truly ignorant and almost superstitious we are in protecting "establishment" Authoritarianism.

Vitamin C in large dosages will not cure Rheumatoid Disease, but it will sure make life easier — and protect your body while doing so!

Chapter XVI
Where Else Does One Look?

In addition to the intraneurals recommended by our treatment protocol, there is increasing interest in the clinical use of lasers for treating neuromata that have been injured. Laser application is much the same as our intraneural treatment except that the skin is not penetrated with a needle, the amplified infra-red providing its own healing effects as it "sees" through the skin.

Anthony Lazzarino D.P.M. of Lewiston, NY has worked with "cold" laser applications to good effect. As a podiatrist he limits himself to lower extremities and the hands, but by the theory of intraneurals he finds himself quite often treating extensive neuro-muscular skeletal systems to relieve patients of pain and symptoms.

A number of our referral physicians are familiar with laser treatments for these purposes.

Other devices, such as neural stimulators, are also in use by various physicians, and warrant investigation by you, if necessary.

Dimethylsulfoxide, known as DMSO, is a by-product of the paper-pulp industry. It is exceedingly cheap and is an extremely good, safe free-radical scavenger. DMSO has had many research papers covering its effects, and there are so many popularized books on the subject that I won't do other than sketch out its major importance to arthritics.

Most all of us who are arthritics have been exposed to the external (and sometimes internal) use of DMSO at one time or another in seeking pain relief.

It has been banned from easy access for our use because "it might be unsafe," yet there is no proof of such unsafety on humans in any properly done research papers.

Arthritics sometimes purchase DMSO from veterinarian suppliers, where it is frequently used for animal pain. Food stores actively promote its sale, and I want to caution you on one deception I encountered.

When the store set on its shelves DMSO with a label stating that it was 90% DMSO "not for human use", I found that the way in which the "90%" was derived was by this means: they decanted DMSO from a large bottle marked as "90% DMSO" filling a small container 10% full of the 90% DMSO and the remainder of the container about 90% full of water.

I leave to first year algebra students the task of determining what the real reduced percentage was!

DMSO when used for arthritis will surely relieve some pain at least temporarily — and in my opinion probably does so with much more safety than would be the taking of aspirin or NSAIDs (non-steroidal anti-inflammatories)

Two books that I recommend for your reading pleasure are: *The Persecuted Drug: The Story of DMSO* by Pat McGrady, Sr. and, Mildred Miller's *A Little Dab Will Do Ya! DMSO: The Drug of the 80's.*

Within these two books, and others on the market, are reports of so many positive features of DMSO that these pages are not adequate to report them all.

Besides being a very good anti-oxidant — free-radical scavenger — it "potentiates" (magnifies) the activity of other medicines, so that you do not need to take as much in order to produce the same results.

If a person who suffers from a very recent cerebral stroke is immediately injected with DMSO (in brain tissue near the hemorrhage) the stroke victim will most likely not be paralyzed or lose powers of speech. The reason: because leaking blood oxidizes to destroy brain neurons (nerve tissue), whereas the DMSO safely anti-oxidizes the leaking blood, thus protecting the neurons from damage. I have known two physicians who have used this method, and have succeeded in bringing about healthy post-stroke victims. Unfortunately most physicians would be too frightened to try this!

DMSO is also used intravenously for a multiplicity of reasons, very much like EDTA, but for different effects. It potentiates the use of EDTA in the veins while also contributing its own good effects, allowing one to use less EDTA — or to achieve "stronger" EDTA action over less time.

When used with and without EDTA it has brought about healing of kidney tissues in patients who've been on continuing dialysis.

DMSO when used intravenously, of course, must be quite pure, not laced with resins and by-products of the wood-pulp industry, and should be buffered with something like potassium carbonate.

There is also strong evidence that it will change rapidly, and safely the ratio of High Density Lipids (HDL) to Low Density Lipids (LDL). I've had one personal experience to verify this through laboratory tests, but I could not answer as to the effect's permanency. One of these lipids is responsible for carrying fats to the cells, and the other one for stuffing the fats in the cells, so to speak, and it always made good sense to me that the ratios ought to be close to one. Young people show an HDL to LDL ratio greater than one. Old folks show a ratio much less than one. My measured ratio was close to that of seventy year men, yet, at the time, I was but 58. After nine IV treatments of DMSO taken three times a week in increasingly stronger dosages, over increasingly long periods of time, my ratio reversed to that of twenty year olds. Multi-vitamins and EDTA did not do this, as I also kept track of my ratio through such treatments to determine exactly what would happen.

Was the treatment beneficial?

I believe it was, but I have no proof to offer, good or

bad.

I've spoken of depression and lethargy that comes with arthritis and continual pain. These symptoms cause mood changes that can from time to time become virtually suicidal, as any arthritic will testify. That some of us do not suicide speaks to the tenacity of life, the love of supporting friends and relatives, and the often abiding faith we have in God.

One medicine that can help us ride through this period, and one that is normally quite safe, is Dilantin, also known as diphenylhydantoin.

Dilantin is also a potentiator of other medicines, but more importantly, it acts to stabilize brain cells into a normalcy of behavior. It is not a narcotic, not addictive, not a stimulant, not a barbiturate, nor is it a tranquilizer. It does little else but permit the brain cells to operate the way they were intended to do.

On taking it you will most probably find that your moods and ability to confront the emotional problems of life increase tremendously. Do not be dissuaded by those who argue that the *Physician's Desk Reference* lists Dilantin for use with epileptics and the brain damaged. There are many, many more uses for Dilantin than reported in that compendium of drug package inserts. Read the book *A Remarkable Medicine Has Been Overlooked* by Jack Dreyfus.

Naturally this chapter is not complete, nor can it be. There are simply too many treatments of a beneficial or possibly beneficial nature, that exist "out there", and if you are to get well, you must take the bull by the horns, so to speak, and begin searching and applying them, preferably with your family physician's active support.

This book had the purpose of informing you, a

victim of Rheumatoid Disease, alternative routes to recovering life without pain, and a future that you will want to live and to enjoy. I cannot promise you that all described will work for you, or that any of it will.

I have, I hope, shown you that establishment-type medicine, with its head-in-the-sand attitude will not accomplish wellness — but you already knew that or you wouldn't be searching still.

The fact that you search still is a very good sign, as it means that you, at least, are open to new and creative ideas — and that's the very first step toward wellness!

If nothing else, I hope you understand that "out there," in alternative medicine land, lies a tremendous number of procedures and techniques and treatment protocols, among which will be one or more that suit you perfectly. Eight out of ten arthritics will get well, or greatly improved through following The Rheumatoid Disease Foundation's suggestions. If your immunological system has already been permanently damaged by dangerous, ineffective establishment-type treatments, there is still hope, for at least 50% of such will be greatly improved or cured. The balance who are not helped should concentrate even harder on those other adjunctive and alternative remedies in this book, and perhaps search for some not as heartily recommended. I will add numerous suggestions shortly.

I can think, for example, of a number of treatments that we do not have room to describe, such as hydrogen peroxide therapy, taken by IV drip.

Macrophages kill invading organisms. With the weakening of the immunological system comes invaders: viral, bacterial, fungal and yeast and mycoplasmas. Your body loses its ability to destroy these invaders by means of peroxides and superoxides produced by macrophages. Apparently hydrogen peroxide therapy provides the missing killing ingredient, peroxides, so that these organisms can be killed in large masses.

Many claims are and have been made about the dangers of this approach, but those who've tried it assure me that it was beneficial to them, and not dangerous at all.

One of our former referral scientists, J. Rinse, Ph.D., suggests that arthritics check into the use of "natural" (unpasteurized, unstrained) honey. He reports on an article by Charles Mraz in *Health Freedom News*, August 1987). Mraz states that natural honey contains dextrose and levulose in about equal proportions.

According to Mraz: Levulose in honey is hygroscopic, it has a great affinity for water so that it can absorb moisture from bacteria in contact with honey and dehydrate them. However, this is not its main bacterial action. Natural honey, also contains an enzyme, 'glucose oxidase'. This enzyme has the interesting activity to take the energy from the honey to produce about 35 parts per million hydrogen peroxide when the honey is diluted.

If honey is heated above about 100 degrees F, this will destroy the action of the enzyme, as will filtering of the honey. This enzyme action of the honey is preserved in that it is not activated until the honey is diluted. As long as the honey is stored in the honey combs, or stored in jars or other containers without any destructive processing this glucose oxidase enzyme remains ready to produce the health giving H_2O_2 just as soon as it is consumed by the bees, and humans that add moisture to it as it is eaten.

The interesting beneficial action of H_2O_2 in honey is, that this action is carried out all through the digestive system of the body. Ordinary "commercial" hydrogen peroxide would be active when first consumed, but the nascent oxygen is released long before it reaches the lower intestines. The enzyme in the honey will continue to produce hydrogen peroxide all through the intestines as long as moisture is added to the honey all during its travel through the digestive system.

I have not investigated this approach, and I would advise caution if you suffer from Candidiasis, as honey contains yeast nutritients: sugar. However, if the effects are what is reported from the peroxides, then it must be through the action of killing off various yeast/fungus, mycoplasmas and other non- natural intestinal microflora. It may be worth a long-term trial.

Oxygen in the form of ozone is provided through IVs in some clinics. Ozone therapy, treating blood externally or internally through complex IV procedures, is used in some foreign countries, also to good effects on various diseases. One of our former referral physicians in West Germany, Helmut Christ M.D. spoke at our Second National Medical Seminar telling us both of his use of ozone therapy as well as a new treatment for Psoriasis that he has found 100% successful on every patient. Such a huge success percentage is unheard of (and almost unbelievable) in medical treatments.

The story is told that Christ's physician friend with Psoriasis himself, tried many different treatments until he stumbled on the use of fumaric acid ester (not fumaric acid!). Apparently the Psoriasis victim's skin lacks fumaric acid ester, or the products with fumaric acid ester. When Helmut Christ obtained the knowledge he was a general practitioner, and had no desire to specialize in Psoriasis. He used the fumaric acid ester "recipes" on several of his patients, and lo! they were healed. Through word of mouth his patients were sending more and more Psoriasis patients to him, and he woke up one morning finding himself, really against his ambition, a specialist in Psoriasis.

A light case of Psoriasis is treated with fumaric acid ester salve, and provided with certain vitamins and minerals. A moderate case may be given fumaric acid ester capsules, and a heavy case the fumaric acid ester capsules, salves and fumaric acid ester soaks, all with various vitamins and minerals.

One caution: while many in the U.S. have had similar results to Christ's patients, I did talk to one lady who could not get these results. Was she treated incorrectly?

Did she really have Psoriasis? Were there complicating factors consisting of other metabolic and/or nutritional and/or disease factors? Is the treatment less than 100% effective?

Live cell therapy is also administered in foreign countries. The theory is that as we age, or sicken, or the endocrine system no longer furnishes us with appropriate substances, by mincing up the proper cells containing these substances from embryos of certain animals, our organs can be revitalized, thus restore the ability to better fight off stress and disease.

True?

I don't know.

Some physicians specialize in the rebalancing of hormones, and seem to have great success in eliminating various diseases, including Rheumatoid Disease. There is no special protocol, but rather an evaluation from day to day of patient needs — and these must be coupled with other good health rules.

A number of good alternative medicine periodicals will keep you abreast of various alternative treatments, and they will often discuss the pros and cons of these treatments so that you are free to form an independent judgment, unbiased by Authority or prejudice, or the strappings of past customs.

Among them is *Medical Hypothesis* available through various libraries, but can also be ordered. Warning: it is written for physicians and scientists, but otherwise very excellent for new ideas.

Townsend Letter for Doctors can be ordered by writing 911 Tyler Street, Port Townsend, WA 98368.

While it is somewhat off the subject, two pamphlets perhaps of interest to you for general information available at The Rheumatoid Disease Foundation: are *Historical Documents In Search of the Cure for Rheumatoid Disease* (ISBN: 0-931150-18-3) with articles by Jack M. Blount, M.D., Archimedes Concon, M.D., James Rowland, D.O., William Renforth, M.D., Paul Williamson, M.D. and Roger Wyburn-Ma- son, M.D. *Dedication, Love and Humour* written by Roger Wyburn-Mason's loving wife, Joan (ISBN: 0-931150-18-3) who describes briefly her life with Professor Roger Wyburn-Mason, the genius who first discovered the effects of medicines in our treatment protocol on Rheumatoid Disease.

The Rheumatoid Disease Foundation is not bound by any treatment, including its own. We do not stand or fall on particular treatments, but rather on accomplishing the goal of eradicating Rheumatoid Diseases.

When a new treatment comes along that is superior in accomplishing this goal, we expect to be in the forefront of its acceptance.

Together you and I have embarked upon a great, if not

grand, adventure, and we want everyone to participate. There are a multitude of ways by which each can contribute, whether by personal services, the setting up of chapters, educating the public and news media, or contributing generously with your limited funds.

One of the most exciting concepts yet unresearched for clinical applications of medicine lies in the field of cell-wall deficient bacteria. Whenever antibiotics are used, various species of bacteria have their walls stripped off in whole or in part. Some of these organisms, instead of dying, revert to a form that can live in body tissue (blood cells) without a wall. It happens that the way in which our immunological system recognizes a foreign invader is through sensing the molecules of the invader's walls. Without a wall, the bacteria cannot be sensed by our immunological system and has protected itself, and it continues to survive. Some bacteria can revert to a viral size and appear to be gone entirely. Later, it can reconstruct itself into common and well known bacteria, and again create the disease — which is our response to its newly grown cell wall. Cell-wall deficient organisms have been known for years, but very little is known about treating them, or how they affect us.

It is research on promising subjects like this that needs your interest and active, willing support. All arthritics will be most grateful — all arthritics worldwide — and all of their arthritic neighbors and relatives — and all of their friends, everywhere!

Meanwhile, please also remember our joint goal. First get yourself well, then your relatives and friends, and afterward help us to go out into the world and eliminate the great crippler!

With great appreciation, I remain, Anthony di Fabio

— but I won't leave you without adding the causations of rheuamatoid disease learned since 1982.

Keep in mind the principle that the human body has but limited ways to response to various stimuli — and it is those stimuli which must be investigated if we're to get and stay well. Here, then, are the factors to investigate. Only a handful of factors will apply to some, but for others, all factors must be investigated!

How Do I Cure
My Rheumatoid Arthritis?
1. How Do I Cure My Rheumatoid Disease?

You start the cure by learning what Rheumatoid Disease is and where it's located in the body and what causes it. The very first thing to learn is that it is a disease of the whole body, not of your joints. This is true no matter how much your joints ache or how insistent is your friendly neighborhood rheumatologist.

2. Where is Rheumatoid Disease Located in my body?

Rheumatoid Disease is a "systemic" disease. This means that whatever ails you is actually a problem of your whole body — cells, organs, systems — the whole works. If you suffer from Rheumatoid Arthritis, for example, this systemic disease is manifesting itself in your joints. If you suffer from a differently named Rheumatoid Disease, then the target area of your body is given a new name, one different from Rheumatoid Arthritis. In fact, there are about 100 differently named diseases that have essentially the same causes but are known under totally different names as shown at the "Articles" tab, "Arthritis Classifications" at our website http://www.arthritistrust.org.

One of our founders, Professor Roger Wyburn-Mason, M.D., Ph.D., explained this astounding fact by describing the medical profession's past technique for naming tuberculosis before discovery of the tuberculin germ. There were about 100 unique names for apparently different diseases depending upon the part of the body affected. Once the tuberculin bacillus was discovered, all of those names collapsed into TB of the bone, TB of the lung, TB of the skin, and so on.

We think Rheumatoid Disease is a cluster of symptoms named differently — 100 unique names — that can now be understood from the viewpoint of a single, systemic disease. (See "Arthritis Classifications" tab at http://www.arthritistrust.org.)

3. But what about my immune system? My doctor says that Rheumatoid Arthritis (or Rheumatoid Disease) is caused by a defective immune system?

There may be some folks who have a defective immune system, but these are probably rare. We believe that your immune system is doing exactly what it was constructed to do. By analogy, consider the camel with too many straws on its back. If you remove those straws one or two at a time eventually the camel will be able to stand again. Our recommended treatment protocol does exactly that — removes the stressors from your immune system until your body (and immune system) functions properly again.

Professor Roger Wyburn-Mason again constructed a useful analogy citing past medical history. Prior to the discovery of the syphilis spirochete, the disease of syphilis was often considered a "defective immune system" disease. It displayed all of the characteristics of an immune system gone awry. Once the spirochete was found it was clear to all that this was an infectious disease problem.

Current internal medicine books will often provide two hypotheses for the cause of Rheumatoid Disease: (a) Something is wrong with the immune system, the body is attacking itself; (b) There is one or more microorganisms inside the body producing a reaction on the rheumatoid disease victim's tissues, thus causing the manifestation of the disease.

Billions of dollars worth of research following up the "something is wrong with the immune system" has never produced a cure. Whereas tens of thousands of arthritics — stemming from the 1960s — have gotten well following up on the second, that is that the body is responding to one or more microorganisms.

4. What microorganism causes this terrible disease? Is there only one that affects everyone the same?

When we started the Arthritis Trust of America (The Rheumatoid Disease Foundation) in 1982 we believed that there was but one nasty microorganism, an amoeba. This was according to the findings of Professor Roger Wyburn-Mason, M.D., Ph.D. and a world-class amoebologist, Dr. Stamm. Dr. Wyburn-Mason was convinced because his treatment designed on the basis of their alleged amoebic findings worked in the large majority of cases. We conducted numerous studies coming at last to the realization that Dr. Wyburn-Mason's treatment protocol was indeed working, but that his belief in an amoebic origin was not necessarily the best answer. (See *The Causation of Rheumatoid Disease and Many Human Cancers*, on Kindle or Nook.)

Meanwhile, independently, Thomas McPherson

Brown, M.D. had concluded that a mycoplasm was the culprit in the creation of Rheumatoid Disease. (See "Thomas McPherson Brown, M.D. Treatment of Rheumatoid Disease," at "Articles Important" tab of http://www.arthritistrust.org.)

There are treatments predicated on both of these hypothesis, except that we've added additional, necessary wellness-serving treatment protocols. These are the necessity of correcting nutritional intake, Candidiasis, food allergies, root canal infections, mercury toxification, herbicide and pesticide accumulations, hormone balancing, and so on.

We now believe that Rheumatoid Disease is caused by many factors (multi-factored) and that there can be one or more out of tens of thousands of invasive microorganisms to which a genetically sensitive person's tissues will respond — either to the microorganisms' protein products or to their waste products. This is known as a "genetic susceptibility" to the toxins or protein products of the microorganism.

5. Should I have tests for these microorganisms, these pathogens?

Unless a health professional has some reason to search for a particular pathogen we feel it is a waste of money and time looking for any specific invader by the taking of blood tests or other traditional tests designed to find pathogens. However, Computerized Electrodermal Screening or kinesiology are two low-cost, often accurate means for making such a determination, if you wish to make the effort.

Experience has shown, however, that broad-spectrum anti-microorganism treatment, coupled with investigation of all the other known causes and assisting treatments, is usually successful, at least 80% of the time.

Here's an example of a patient where our recommended anti-microorganism drugs did not work, but, by following our principles, the patient recovered from Ankylosing Spondilitis, one of the 100 or so named Rheumatoid Diseases. Reason: he was exposed to a whole different type of invading microorganism than normally found in the United States, *Schistosomiasis bilharzia*, a parasite obtained by swimming in Zimbabwe waters at an altitude where the waters are known to harbor this organism. He was able to get well by using the proper pharmaceutical created for this specific microorganism together with proper application of our other treatment recommendations — that is, unloading the immune system. (See http://www.arthritistrust.org, "Newsletters" "Spring 2005.")

We know patients who achieved wellness using only our recommended anti-microorganism treatments.

We also know of patients who only needed our other recommendations — not the anti-microorganism protocol — and got well.

Some patients require many or all of our recommendations to achieve wellness.

But, concentrate on the principles we describe and not on a literal-minded authoritarian approach.

6. How will I know exactly what to do? Take the anti-microorganism treatment or the other treatments?

Your best bet — if you truly want to get well — is to work with one or more knowledgeable health professional, and to remove every single suppressor, every straw on the camel's back! You must learn more than your friendly neighborhood rheumatologist. This will be easy to do, because this group of professionals know absolutely nothing about how to get you well (according to their own statements), and you'll know something!

One drawback is this: There's no one health professional or dentist in the United States who offers all the treatment recommendations you will need to explore. Several clinics come close, but the majority of those who signed up on our physician referral list in the past were rather limited in what they chose to offer you. So, if you truly want to get well, you should consider several options right at the start.

a. First off, learn everything you can on this website. Especially read the book *Arthritis* by Prosch and di Fabio at Kindle and Nook.

If you don't understand some of the words, use "Google" or a dictionary or some other search engine to define them. Don't let words stand between you and a good understanding of the principles for achieving wellness. You won't have to learn your friendly neighborhood rheumatologist's complex medical language, thank goodness, but you'll need to clear up some basic concepts to avoid confusion.

b. After you've learned as much as you feel you can absorb, then start searching for a health professional who will work with you. This could be your family doctor. We'll help her/him to learn, if s/he is open-minded and willing to learn.

Otherwise, you can search for a doctor in your geographical region who is dedicated to or inclined to practice alternative/complementary medicine. All of our past referral doctors categorized themselves as alternative/complementary doctors, but they individually restrict themselves to specialty treatment protocols only some of which remove straws from the camel's back.

Plan on traveling to another location where exists a health professional who will help — and then plan on traveling to another location to visit another health professional. You will understand this option better when you go over the causes of arthritis, and removal of the straws in the instructions that follow.

By now you're thinking, "Good gosh! This is getting complicated. I only want a pill to make me feel better and to get me well."

That's the kind of thinking encouraged by your present treatment plan, and the very reason that you're not getting well. It's an "authoritarian" approach. Face it! There's no pill that will remove all the straws from the camel's back.

There may be easier ways for achieving wellness, and if you find them, please let us know so we can tell others. Meanwhile, here's our recommended treatment protocol!

7. Proper Nutrition is important! So what is proper nutrition for the Arthritic?

There are numerous animal and plant substances considered to be "food" around the world. No one country has a monopoly on what is right, or even what is right for you.

Regardless of your genetic background, native country, religious bent, or family tradition, you must find a way to change your diet so that your tissues are primarily alkaline rather than acidic. What you eat determines this situation!

To be sure that you're capable of utilizing the nutrients that you take in through the mouth, some physicians will want to test the acidity of your stomach. They'll want to know, "Are you actually absorbing your food?" If not, they'll place you on a proper regimen to handle this common problem. (The stomach is one place that you want acidity. Read Dr. Wright's "Myth of Acid Indigestion — Heartburn & GERD" at http:www.arthritistrust.org under the "Articles Important" tab.)

The health professional may also want to know if your metabolism is capable of operating at the correct rate. Without a proper overall metabolic temperature, essential enzymes will not chemically unfold to manipulate your digested and absorbed nutrients. If low, you'll probably need thyroid supplements — but only the right kind, not the generally administered type given out by traditional medical practitioners. Read "Thyroid Hormone Therapy: Cutting the Gordian Knot" at http:www.arthritistrust.org under the ""Articles Important" tab.

Assuming all the other hormones are functioning properly, then the general dietary principle is simple, but requires a definition of "food," which we now provide.

There are two types of things routinely placed in folks' mouths. One is called "food" and the other is called "non-food." So that you'll better understand "food" we'll first define "non-food."

"Non-food" is everything you place in your mouth that has been packaged, processed, treated, frozen, or otherwise stabilized for long grocery store shelf life.

"Food" is what you get out of the garden, or from the animals that have provided meat that is fresh, untainted, and untreated.

The closer you can eat from the garden (or killed animal) the healthier. Similarly, the further away from the garden (or killed animal) you eat, the unhealthier — especially when your intake derives from substances packaged, processed, treated, frozen, or otherwise stabilized for long grocery store shelf life.

Some call this the "cave-man" diet. But you don't have to be a cave-man as the principles are really not that difficult to follow.

One exception to the "food" vs. "non-food" designation and restriction on "non-foods" is your liberal use of proper supplements. Your friendly neighborhood rheumatologist may tell you that these are simply "expensive urine." Don't disturb her/his authoritarian fantasies! There are very good reasons why properly prepared and packaged vitamins, minerals and essential fatty acids are absolutely essential for your wellness trek, and in any case, the lack of some of these may be weighty straws holding down the camel's back.

For excellent descriptions of appropriate Rheumatoid Disease diets, read the following articles on our website at http://www.arthritistrust.org, under the "Articles Important" tab: "Natural Treatment for Arthritis," Proper Nutrition for Rheumatoid Arthritis," and "The Perfect Health Plan."

8. It's important that I check out Candidiasis Infection. So what is it?

You must determine if you've got systemic Candidiasis infection and, if so, you must get rid of the infection.

Many excellent books have been written on this subject. We'll not repeat the great deal known about this modern plague, but we'll cover some important essentials.

Candida albicans — among other invasive organisms-of-opportunity — is a yeast/fungus with at least six known "switching mechanisms." A "switching mechanism" is simply a microorganism's method of survival. When the environment is changed surrounding it — say from acid to alkaline, for example — the microorganism switches to a different form and function, one that permits it to survive in the new environment.

Candida albicans (among other invasive organisms) has one very nasty switching mechanism that spreads throughout the intestinal tract, also pushing or growing a "rootlet" right thru your protective intestinal mucosa. This opening permits undigested molecular-sized proteins to go directly into your blood stream where your ever-watchful immune system spots it, recognizes that protein molecule as an invader (antigen), and proceeds to construct an antibody to protect you from it. This "antigen/ antibody" relationship results in an increasing number of food allergies.

Food allergies not only produce their own unique health problems, but can also mimic most of the degenerative diseases, including Rheumatoid Diseases.

Candidiasis also results in a yeast production of either alcohol or acetylhyde, the metabolite of alcohol. Acetylhyde is believed to be the part that gives you a hang-over after drinking too much alcohol the night before.

Constant, persistent production of these products, even at a low level, not only create their own special health problems, but can also mimic many of the degenerative diseases.

Some physicians estimate that about 50% of their Rheumatoid Disease patients suffer from Candidiasis. Other physicians estimate a higher rate. We've known one friendly neighborhood rheumatologist to pronounce a patient who suffered only from Candidiasis as having Rheumatoid Arthritis, and proceeded thereafter to prescribe the standard, non-effective and damaging methotrexate. Of course, the patient did not get well for two reasons: (1) She didn't have Rheumatoid Arthritis in the first place; and, (2) Methotrexate at best covers up arthritic symptoms while permitting the disease to rage onward.

The main reason for this pathetic mistake is that traditional medical practitioners do not accept systemic candidiasis as a commonly acquired disease!

So where do folks acquire Candidiasis?

There are several main direct routes to its being acquired: (a) Use of antibiotics administered by medical practitioners for an infection kill off the "good-guys'" intestinal microflora and permits organisms-of-opportunity to flourish; (b) Long stretches of stress brings on their intestinal overburdening; (c) The use of the immune suppressing drugs against Rheumatoid Disease (or other disease states) brings on the overgrowth.

So — you must understand — that the very drugs that you've been given by your friendly neighborhood rheumatologist, or your family general practitioner, may have created the unwanted overgrowth. At the very least, it helps this nasty growth to survive.

There are numerous solutions to Candidiasis, some better than others. Read "Candidiasis: Scourge of Arthritics," at http://www.arthritistrust.org under the "Articles Important" tab. Here you'll find that a blood test sent to the proper laboratory can determine infestation, but that normally the health professional will rely on your answers to a specially designed questionaire, as well as other signs and symptoms. The referenced article contains such a questionaire one used by Gus J. Prosch, Jr., M.D. for his patients.

You must rid yourself of Candidiasis for many

reasons, least of which is that it could be the actual source of your Rheumatoid Disease symptoms. If not the source, then certainly it will be a contributing factor — one of the camel's straws!

By the way, for females, a vaginal infection is generally symptomatic of a systemic infection. Treating only the vagina, as recommended by standard medical advice, is not the general, systemic solution!

9. It's vital that I spot and handle my food allergies. So, how do I do this?

Food allergies may be one of the most common reasons for the manifestation of many kinds of degenerative disease, including Rheumatoid Disease. You've already read how Candidiasis can promote food allergies, but food allergies can also occur in other ways.

One of the most surprising — and distasteful — facts about food allergies is that allergies' biological rules are virtually the same as those of drug addiction! A person called an "alcoholic" has a "food" allergy. S/he's allergic to alcohol!

We "like" and always eat certain foods because we're addicted to them!

We develop food allergies from (a) "foods" most easily digested and assimilated, and (b) those "foods" eaten most often; i.e., the "foods" we really like.

"Foods" that are most easily digested and assimilated are, in their order of ease (a) alcohol, (b) sugar, (c) simple carbohydrates like white flour and products made with white flour, and rice.

Complex carbohydrates, such as whole vegetables, and various proteins from meats are not so easily digested and assimilated, but can also be a source of food allergies, especially if eaten regularly, i.e., daily or near daily; or, if systemic Candidiasis is present most any food can be allergenic.

Warren Levin, M.D. explains the food allergy (drug addiction) phenomena very nicely at http://www.arthritistrust.org at the "Articles Important" tab in his "Allergies and Biodetoxification for the Arthritic." He also provides a 5-day abstinence fasting program together with the keeping of a food intake and symptom log that assists in determining exactly what foods create a problem for you. (Some foods cause reactions immediately while others require three days to kick in, thus, the need for a written calendar "food" intake log.)

William H. Philpott, M.D. also provides a solution to the food allergy problem through the use of benign heavy-duty magnets and a 5-day or 7-day food rotation diet. Go to http://www.arthritistrust.org, "Research" thence to "Research and Letters," and then look for his name at the alphabetized list to the left. You'll find many complete articles of Dr. Philpott's describing the beneficial use of heavy-duty magnets and rotation diets for food allergies.

Some "foods," rather than allergenic, are chemically disturbing to people with a genetic susceptibility to those products. Ed Wendlocher and other scientists have determined the source of arthritic pain for many folks as stemming from hot chili peppers, especially those found in various "food" products as flavor enhancers, but not listed on the labels. Go to http://www.arthritistrust.org to the "Articles Important" tab and read his "Chemicals in 'hot' Chili Peppers Confirmed to be a Cause of Arthritis."

Appropriate blood tests from a properly equipped laboratory can also help determine your food allergies;

172

and, it goes without further explanation that those well trained and experienced in the application of electrodermal screening or kinesiology can also help make this determination.

It's very important that you find your food allergies and that you handle them, especially if the allergies are a component of causation — another straw — for your Rheumatoid Disease!

10. Yes, that's all very well, but what about the anti-microorganism treatment? I want to start with that treatment because I've heard so much about it!

Certainly many more Rheumatoid Arthritis victims have gotten well from anti-microorganism treatment than any other treatment used by the accepted medical establishment. Although some few rheumatologists will try Thomas McPherson Brown's anti-mycoplasm treatment and some few will try the Roger Wyburn-Mason anti-microorganism treatment, the mistake both make is in still subscribing to the archaic nineteenth century philosophy that for each disease there is one microorganism. Kill that organism and wellness ensues. This is true for many infectious diseases, but generally not true for the so-called "degenerative" diseases, which are usually multi-factored — caused by many factors.

Generally, though, your friendly neighborhood rheumatologist will not wander from the path laid down by his peers, his hospital, or insurance providers, none of which achieve wellness, but rather, provide you with damaging drugs that permit you to function without pain a little longer while the crippling disease rages onward.

Please consider this: While some of us have gotten free of Rheumatoid Arthritis simply by taking a drug, failures usually occur because the physician or the patient has ignored the rest of the camel's straws. We know, as fact, that Dr. Gus J. Prosch's consistent arthritic cure rate of 80% occurred because he and the patient also tackled other causations at the same time.

So, when you reach this aspect of your treatment program you've got two choices: (a) the Thomas McPherson Brown anti-mycoplasm approach, or (b) the Roger Wyburn-Mason (the Arthritis Trust of America) broad spectrum anti-microorganism approach.

Frankly, we're not selling either one. We're only interested in your wellness!

And, we've had folks call or write to tell us they've been on one or the other approach, and they're still not well.

Frankly, too, practitioners who subscribe to one approach and not to the other both claim about 80% cure rate, sometimes both sides pooh-poohing the other side.

We do, however, recommend that you start with the Arthritis Trust of America (Wyburn-Mason) approach for several rational reasons:

(a) You'll know in about six to twelve weeks whether or not it will work whereas, for the anti-mycoplasm approach you'll know in about a year. If the arthritis broad spectrum anti-microorganism treatment doesn't work, you can still try the anti-mycoplasm approach. The Arthritis Trust of America recommended anti-microorganism approach taking only six to twelve weeks will then require only about 2 or 3 visits to your assisting health professional. Whereas the anti-mycoplasm approach takes periodic visits for a year.

(b) The Arthritis Trust of America anti-microorganism approach is cheaper.

If you're a gambler, and like to play for the jackpot

with your paycheck, then try either of these without removing the other straws. Either might work without removing the additional straws — but really, now, don't bet too heavily on it!

11. What is the Arthritis Trust of America anti-microorganism approach?

With some modification by a committee of our referral physicians, it's the same as the Professor Roger Wyburn-Mason, M.D., Ph.D. development begun in the 1960s. He was curing patients worldwide. We'll list the main ingredients here, but for a complete picture go to http://www.arththritistrust.org, the "Articles Important" tab, and find "Wyburn-Mason Treatment for Rheumatoid Disease." (You may also go to Kindle or Nook and find a detailed description of this anti-microorganism treatment in each of the books: *Rheumatoid Disease Cured at Last*, *The Art of Getting Well*, *Little Known Treatments for Arthritis*, and *Arthritis: Osteoarthritis and Rheumatoid Disease Including Rheumatoid Arthritis*. In particular, for health professionals, please also read *Causation of Rheumatoid Disease: and Many Human Cancers*.)

Recommended broad spectrum prescription drugs are the following:

(a) Metronidazole - Get from any pharmacy.

(b) Clotrimazole - Get through a compounding pharmacist.

(c) Tinidazole - Get through a compounding pharmacist, except in the American Southwest get from most pharmacies.

(e) Nimorazole - Cannot get in the United States.

(f) Ornidazole - Cannot get in the United States.

Above (a) thru (f) are called the 5-nitroimidazoles.

(g) Allopurinol - Get from any pharmacy.

(h) Furazolidone - Get from any pharmacy.

Here's how they are used to make up a <u>broad-spectrum</u> anti-microorganism treatment:

First, your health professional must be assured that your liver and kidneys can tolerate these drugs in the dosage prescribed. The dosage recommended is by body weight. Do not permit your doctor to lower the dosage below the recommended body weight simply because he thinks you cannot tolerate the drugs. If you can't tolerate the drugs, don't take any of them!

Baseline is 200 pounds. If you weigh 200 pounds, then you should take two grams (2000 mgs) of one of the drugs "a" thru "f" each day for two days in a row, like, for example, Saturday and Sunday. Then you skip taking any drugs for five days, a drug washout period. Then you take 2 grams (2000 mgs) per day for two successive days the next Saturday and Sunday. In all, you repeat this process for six weeks.

During the first seven days you also take 300 mg of allopurinol (item "g") 3 times a day, each day. Then stop! No more allopurinol for this cycle of treatment!

If for some odd reason you're allergic to allopurinol, or your health professional thinks s/he would prefer to have you do so, then take furazolidone (item "h") for the first 10 successive days, 100 mg 3 times per day. Then stop. No more furazolidone for this cycle of treatment!

Important: For each 25 pounds over or under the 200 pound baseline that you weigh, you either add or substract 250 mg (1/4 gram), respectively, to the 5-nitroimidazole prescription.

Some doctors since 1982 have varied this standardized protocol with success. For example, Gus J.

176

Prosch, Jr., M.D. often tried a second cycle of treatments using a different one of the 5-nitroimidazoles. John Parks Trowbridge, M.D. developed a slightly different protocol with success, and he added in the use of DHEA/ pregnenolone IV (intravenous natural hormone replacement) plus EDTA chelation IV, whence usually 80-90% are helped. He also monitors blood tests. (Press the tab "Articles Important," and go to the article "Chelation Therapy," on our website http://www.arthritistrust.org for the nature of EDTA chelation IV; and also for "Hormone Balancing: Natural Treatment & Cure for Arthritis.")

It bears repetition! The principles of treatment are important, not the literal-minded interpretation of rules!! If your health professional and you get good results, then both of you know what you're doing!!!

12. My doctor says that metronidazole might cause cancer. Is this correct?

Metronidazole is not carcinogenic. This is one of the most popular discreditations, unrelated to fact. According to a Senator Ted Kennedy joint hearing before the subcommittee on labor and public welfare and the subcommittee on administrative practice and procedure of the committee on the *Judiciary United States Senate Ninety Fourth Congress, July 10, 11, 1975*, Searle (pharmaceutical company) representatives testified that some lab data had been misplaced regarding control group rats, and that carcinogenic symptoms had been observed *in the control group* (the rat group that was not on metronidazole). The FDA, they said, had required them to throw the carcinogenic count into the non control group. [See "First Session On Examination of the Process of Drug Testing and FDA's Role in the Regulation and Conditions Under Which Such Testing is Carried Out,"

Preclinical and clinical testing by the Pharmaceutical Industry, 1975, Published by the U.S. Government Printing Office, Washington, D.C. 1975]

Thus, the *Physicians Desk Reference* now contains the statement that metronidazole may cause cancers in rats. This error has never been corrected on a drug package insert, and probably never will be.

In an address by Wayne Martin [deceased] of Fairhope, Alabama, before the Seattle Chapter of the International Association of Cancer Victims and Friends, he summarized the results of a study of Flagyl (metronidazole) in the treatment of cancer:

In the Seattle area, the Group Health Cooperative of Puget Sound has treated 12,280 patients with Flagyl (metronidazole) mostly for the parasitic disease trichomonoasis, which causes urogenital distress. Of this group, only five patients developed cancer over a 2-1/2 year period, whereas among the 123,620 non Flagyl users, 311 patients developed cancer over the same period of time. On a percentage basis, 0.04% of the Flagyl patients developed cancer, compared with 2.5% of the non Flagyl users — a score of better than 60 to 1 in favor of Flagyl users. When a correction for age was factored in, the score was still 3 to 1 in favor of Flagyl users *(Journal of the American Medical Association,* May 14, 1982, pp. 2498 2499.)

The *Physicians Desk Reference* also states that since 1967 there has never been a reported case of human carcinogenicity or mutagenicity through the use of metronidazole.

According to *The First Metronidazole Conference,* metronidazole is world widely used, often in dosages much higher than our recommendations, and often in hospital settings where it is frequently used intravenously in very high dosages for bacterial infections.

13. My doctor uses intravenous metronidazole in hospitals to kill bacteria. He says he's willing to give me the same treatment since he knows it's safe. Should I use it?

Intravenous dosages of metronidazole will do nothing to halt the progress of Rheumatoid Disease, although it might ease the free radical damage for a short time. Reason: Your "good-guys" microflora must "metabolize" the drug. It's the metabolites of metronidazole that kill the microorganisms, not the drug itself. Your "good-guys" microflora should be supplemented with a good quality grade of supplemental *Lactobaccilus acidophilus* & *Bifido bacterium*. Such supplementation is important for the proper activation of the metronidazole and other 5-nitroimidazoles.

14. What signs and symptoms should my doctor and I look for?

You should both look for the Herxheimer effect!

In 1902 two research physicians, Doctors Adolph Jarisch and Karl Herxheimer, studied the treatment of syphilis, using various kinds of relatively dangerous drugs. They learned that whenever they killed the syphilis spirochete the patient displayed a series of symptoms similar to "flu." They later concluded that whenever an organism more complex than a simple bacteria was killed within the human body, one had these same symptoms. Subsequently this phenomenon became named the "Jarisch-Herxheimer" or "Herxheimer" effect.

When treating tuberculosis, the Herxheimer occurs, as it also does in treating Leishmaniasis. When treating Leprosy, the same phenomenon occurs, but it's called "Lucio's" phenomenon." Some other rare, tropical diseases also exhibit the Herxheimer when treated by killing the causative organism. Some call it the "die off effect" — for example in treating Candidiasis — as it occurs whenever the invading organism is dying off.

According to the Jarisch-Herxheimer theory, when an invading organism (more complex than a simple bacteria) acts as an antigen (allergy agent) the body prepares antibodies that tend to fight the antigen. This creates products which are the cause of the swelling, heat, and joint damage. One's tissues and immune system responds to the killing of the organism inside the body by producing a serious allergic response inside the body. The products of that allergic response create secondary problems that lead to the additional damage.

If there is a causative organism that creates RD, and if the organism is killed by this medicine, and if you've been sensitized to the protein products of that organism, then more of the protein products resulting from dead organisms will increase the internal allergic response. It follows, therefore, that, just by killing off one of the causative agents of Rheumatoid Disease, the body will have an intensification of the very symptoms that we label as "Rheumatoid Disease." Rheumatoid Disease symptoms are a systemic manifestation of the internal allergy!

The Herxheimer effect consists of these signs and symptoms:

(a.) General and usual: Sweating and especially night sweats, diarrhea, nausea, vomiting, headache, fever, general malaise, flushing of skin, anorexia, aching bones and "flu" symptoms resembling a serum reaction.

(b.) The inflamed and affected tissues become

more inflamed and tissues previously unknown to be involved become inflamed.

(c.) If the heart, pericardium or cardiac tissues are infected, patients may develop some paroxysmal auricular tachycardia, premature ventricular contractions or ectopic beats.

(d.) If the urinary bladder tissues are infected the patient may develop signs of full-blown cystitis.

(e.) If the brain or meninges are infected the patient may develop severe (temporary) depression, lethargy, generalized weakness, temporary memory loss, irritability along with headaches.

(f.) If the mouth tissues are infected, a bitter and/or metallic taste may be noted along with mild shedding or peeling of the mucosal tissues. This has also been noted in the rectal tissues. However, it should be noted that Metronidazole and Tinidazole also produce a metallic taste without the Herxheimer effect being present.

(g.) When the periosteal tissues and skeletal muscle tissues are involved, fairly severe bone pain usually accompanied by severe muscle pains and spasms may be observed, usually at night.

(h.) When the lungs and bronchial tissues are infected the patients may develop bronchitis symptoms and occasionally pneumonitis (resembling viral) has been observed.

You and your physician must learn to distinguish between the possible effects of drug toxicity, an allergic reaction to one or more drugs, or the Herxheimer effect. (See http://www.arthritistrust.org, "Articles Important" tab, "The Herxheimer Effect.")

15. What if the Herxheimer effect becomes so

strong that I can't tolerate it?

The Herxheimer is a good sign, because then both you and your doctor know that the drug is killing organisms. Something good is really happening! When your body cleans up the antigen/antibody complexes, you'll probably be free of Rheumatoid Disease — assuming the other straws do not need to be removed.

To tolerate the Herxheimer, when we first designed our treatment protocol in 1982 we made certain recommendations related to the taking of small amounts of prednisone or, perhaps, non-steroidal anti-inflammatory drugs. We don't like what prednisone does to the body, but, if no other recourse is available to you, one of those options may be necessary.

But, what we truly know will work favorably is the judicious application of Dr. Pybus' Intraneural Injections!

What we know about the use of intraneural injections simultaneous with your visit to your doctor fills another booklet, which you'll find at Kindle and Nook also *Intraneural Injections for Rheumatoid Arthritis & Ostoearthritis & Control of Pain in Arthritis of the Knee.*

Indeed, Dr. Prosch's consistent success rate depended upon use of all of the above, including same day use of intraneural injections. The Arthritis Trust of America feels that the booklet, *Intraneural Injections for Rheumatoid Arthritis and Osteoarthritis & The Control of Pain in Arthritis of the Knee,* by Dr. Paul K. Pybus, is a must for all forms of Rheumatoid Disease and arthritis-like pain, and that the use where appropriate of designated intraneural injections decreases the time to wellness, regardless of what other modalities are used on the patient. One important advantage being the ability to get the patient off of damaging pain-relieving drugs while the body is adapting to healing treatments and wellness routines. These easy-to-administer injections address the source of your joint pain, nerve ganglia that lead to the affected joint. (You'll also find a description of Intraneural Injections at http://www.arthritistrust.org, "Newsletters," Spring, Summer, Fall, . . . 2006.)

Englishman Roger Wyburn-Mason, M.D., Ph.D., nerve specialist, was the first to describe the source (not causation) principle of joint damage from tender nerve locations, sometimes called "trigger points," in arthritis and arthritis-like pain.

South African Dr. Paul K. Pybus, his former house physician, learned to implement in clinical practice Wyburn-Mason's theories of intraneural injections, successfully using his discoveries for more than 20 years.

Keith McElroy, M.D. (The New York Orthopaedic Hospital) independently discovered the same principles, and applied them to his patients, also for many years. He called them "Injection Therapy."

Dr. Paul K. Pybus and Gus J. Prosch, Jr., M.D. explored additional key "trigger points," until it became clear to them that a virtual one-to-one correspondence existed between painful neuroma and acupuncture points — but not always so.

Dr. I.H.J. Bourne, a friend of both Dr. Roger Wyburn-Mason and Dr. Paul Pybus, also developed the use of intraneural injections which he published as "Musculoskeletal Disorders: Local Injection Therapy." His paper and Dr. Prosch's has been added to the rear of the aforenoted intraneural injection booklet at Kindle or Nook. *(Intraneural Injections for Rheumatoid Arthritis and Osteoarthritis & The Control of Pain in Arthritis of the Knee*)

Dr. Curt Maxwell of Los Algodones, Mexico uses all injection modalities. While the book does not address itself to inflammed neuroma, he also recommends the W.B. Saunders book, *Atlas of Pain Management Injection Techniques* by Steven D. Waldman, M.D., J.D. as an excellent supplementary book. (It is very convenient for doctors who are into reimbursement via insurance, as it gives the insurance code that is acceptable for each of the injections. The artwork is excellent, and there can be no doubt as to how to do the recommended injections in the various parts of the body. The text is quite appropriate, giving not only the how, but also contra-indications, et. al.)

Of additional major importance, for more than 50 years American Harry H. Philbert, M.D. independently developed the use of what he chose to call "Specific Injection Therapy," covering many of the same aspects as the several intraneural publications reported above. *The Anatomy of Pain: Specific Injection Therapy*, is a well-done report by Dr. Philbert.

To clarify further, your doctor should know how to use any one of several types of injections: (a) Intraneural Injections, (b) Neural Therapy according to Huenke, and (c) Sclerotherapy [Prolo or Proliferative Therapy or Reconstructive Therapy].

Neural Therapy (Injections), developed by Ferdinand and Walter Huenke, also about 70 years ago, addresses the problem of patterns of stored "pain" reflexes which trigger off permanent relief upon injection. These injections are particularly important when addressing scar tissue and the ability of such permanent scars to distort structure.

Sclerotherapy (or Prolo Therapy) is very important for tightening up tendons or ligaments that have become stretched or torn. This eventually applies to all arthritics, but is not germane at this point, except that in any form of arthritis many joint pains do, in fact, stem from stretched or torn ligaments and tendons. This is the only treatment that can permanently solve that problem. (You can read more about it at http://www.arthritistrust.org, "Articles Important" tab, in "Sclero Therapy — Prolo Therapy," and, if you're a health professional, *Structural Diagnostic Photography*, by James A. Carlson, D.O. at Kindle or Nook.)

When using the intraneural injection protocol, your doctor will probably want you to return in about three weeks. That's about the length of time that the effects of the intraneural injections will last, permitting you and your doctor during the interim to work on removing as many of the camel's straws as possible. At that time, you can receive another set of injections which will safely — and almost miraculously — remove your joint pain for another three weeks.

Once you've rid yourself of the Rheumatoid Disease, you may still need some injections, but each time you receive them there'll be less pain points and the injections will last longer. (This aspect is covered in more detail in the aforementioned Dr. Pybus' book on intraneural injections at our website.)

16. What about the Thomas McPherson Brown, M.D. anti-mycoplasm treatment?

This treatment is predicated on the assumption that the mycoplasm is the cause of Rheumatoid Disease and a form of antibiotic is used to kill this microorganism. Treatment is usually spaced out over numerous visits throughout the year. At each visit a small amount of a specific antibiotic is given. This is called "pulsing." For further information go to our website at http://www.arthritistrust.org, "Articles Important" tab, "Thomas McPherson Brown, M.D. Treatment of Rheumatoid Disease."

17. My doctor has done all of the above, and I'm still not well! What do I do next?

Eighty percent of those treated by Dr. Prosch, and other doctors, have gotten well, many for the first time in years of suffering. You must be one among the remaining 20%. Too bad! But don't give up. It simply means that you've got more straws to remove, and it's important that you know what they are, and how to remove them.

In fact, the successful 80% also should be routinely removing these additional straws to continue strengthening their immune system!!

Some remaining important straws are: (a) root canal cleansing, (b) mercury removal, (c) intestinal cleansing, and (d) detoxification.

18. I've taken very good care of my teeth — spent lots of money. I've got a very good dentist and he says that I don't need any further work on my gums or removal of mercury. He says you folks are crazy!

Well, then, I guess you've got a choice! Stay away from crazy people, or get yourself well!

We've learned over the years that it's more difficult to wean Rheumatoid Disease victims away from their very friendly neighborhood dentist than it is from their friendly neighborhood rheumatologist. We can understand the reasons. You've just gone through a stressful series of dental sessions, and you've put out big bucks, and now you might have to do it all over again? Crazy, indeed!

Here's the problem: Whenever root canal work has been completed, or a tooth has been extracted, the dentist is not taught to remove the tough integument that held the tooth in place. This tough tissue keeps antibiotics from getting into the cavitation formed there. Your friendly neighborhood dentist has not been taught this fact, although it was his trade union's predecessors who funded affirming definitive studies on this subject many years ago. Bacteria that lives in your mouth and that has gotten locked into these cavities mutates from an oxygen-loving form (aerobic) to one that does not love oxygen (anaerobic), and sets up shop behind this tough tissue. It begans manufacturing some of the most deadly toxins in the world, ten times more deadly than botulism. Radioactive substances have traced these poisonous toxins to specific organs in the body with resulting disease states.

Only ten percent of folks are aware of having any microbial growth there, so silently do these organisms work — and, through their stealthy action, they also become the source for persistent bone shrinkage as folks age.

Removing this important straw requires a "biological dentist," one who is trained in identifying this kind of problem, and who can safely cleanse the infected cavitation. No matter how kind and friendly your family dentist, s/he will not have been trained in this area, and will most likely pooh pooh the idea!

Again you can rely on non-invasive electro-dermal screening, or kinesiology to make a determination of need for this straw's removal. But in addition, the Biology Department at the University of Kentucky developed a method for the dentist to swab the base of the gums at each tooth and determine whether or not there's an infection in the tooth's root canal.

The Price Pottenger Nutrition Foundation will provide you with names and addresses of biological dentists near you. Caution, however, their list does not show which biological dentists are trained for safe mercury removal and which trained for both cavitation cleansing and safe mercury removal. You'll have to call the various biological dentists and ask.

George E. Meinig, D.D.S., F.A.C.D., one of the nineteen founding members that organized the American Association of Endodontists and a former Twentieth Century Fox Studio dentist, discussed this serious health problem in his book *Root Canal Coverup*.

You should order this book and read it!

19. My dentist says that once mercury has been combined with other metals and placed in my teeth, it's safe and doesn't create any problems. So, why should I redo all that beautiful, expensive workmanship?

Your dentist is demonstrably wrong!

Regardless of which doctor, dentist or organization tells you that mercury is safe once it's placed in your mouth, and saying "it's safe" doesn't make it safe! They're flat out wrong! They haven't done their homework! They're simply repeating a long-standing falsehood!

Let's consider some provable facts:

a. The EPA as well as the American Medical Association states that there is no lower safe limit to the amount of mercury a person can intake.

b. Dentists and their employees are required to handle mercury in special ways that the Environmental Protection Agency considers safe because of mercury's extreme health hazard. This protection is for the benefit of the dentist and her/his employees and their office, not the patient.

c. The two different metals (the amalgam) immersed in an acid or alkaline environment (the mouth) produces an electromotive force which is easily measurable at each filled tooth.

d. This electric current plus the mouth's acidity or alkalinity causes a small amount of the amalgam to vaporize in your mouth. The vapor combines with organic materials to form a very toxic mercury molecule that accumulates in your body.

e. The stored organic mercury compound added to other mercury from the intake of food and from pesticides and herbicides can eventually cause any one of many forms of degenerative disease, including those of Rheumatoid Disease.

f. After many years of resistance, just like the American Dental Association (a protective trade union), the Swedish Dental Association studied the problem, apologized to their citizens, and phased out mercury. Most of the European community has also done so. Only the stubborn, intransigent American Dental Association — probably fearful of expensive accumulating law suits like the tobacco industry — resists.

Three doctors working together in Tijuana, Mexico felt so strongly about the importance of mercury stress on the body that they refused to accept an American Rheumatoid Arthritis patient until he'd cleared his mouth of mercury amalgams through an American biological dentist. Once properly cleared, the American no longer had a need to visit these Mexican doctors as the patient's Rheumatoid Arthritis had magically disappeared!

While perhaps statistically improbable, this true

anecdote nicely illustrates the point of safely removing mercury and other metals from your mouth. We say "safely" because, if you should decide it's more convenient and cheaper to have your friendly neighborhood dentist do the job (if he's willing), you could easily end up sicker than when you started. Why? Because the order in which the amalgams are removed is important, and the manner in which you're protected from mercury fumes while removing the amalgams is paramount.

A "biological" dentist has the tools and know how and is important for your health!

We recommend dentist Hal Huggins' *Uninformed Consent* book.

20. After I've safely removed all the metal in my mouth will that take care of all of my mercury?

Probably not. Your body has taken your lifetime to store up mercury from various sources: teeth, food, vaccination shots (preservatives), pesticides and herbicides that surround us everywhere, to name a few major sources.

There's several means for ridding your body of mercury, each requiring help from a knowledgeable health professional, some taking longer than others.

a. Chelate the mercury from your body using proper chelating agents. Periodic urine and hair samples may assist in determining effectiveness. Repeated visits for some time may be necessary.

b. Use chlorella with your other nutritional supplements. This may take a long time.

c. Use kinesiology and/or electrodermal screening to determine location of mercury accumulation, and then drive the organic mercury out thru use of either (1) magnetic polarity, or (2) injections of novacaine in the mercury deposits. The novacaine converts to a B vitamin that drives the mercury out of nerve ganglia where stored, according to Lee Cowden, M.D.

21. Is colon cleansing really necessary? If so, what do I do?

Detoxification of the body is one of the most neglected wellness projects, although most health professionals realize that a sick body is a toxic one. Some health professionals feel that the colon is one of the most important organs in the body. Here you'll find the source of many diseases, and you'll also find the lack of desirable microorganisms and many unwanted microorganisms: bacterial, viral, amoebic, mycoplasmic, worms, and yeast/fungus infections. Any one of these can create the tissue sensitivity that brings about your arthritic condition. There are numerous methods for ridding your body of these undesirables, or (replacing the desirables) advocated by various health professionals. If your doctor is unversed in colon cleansing, then seek out an alternative/complementary health professional. More than likely one with an N.D. degree (naturopathy) will be knowledgeable in colon cleansing.

Toxic acids are normal products of cell catabolism, and we also take in many toxic products when breathing, eating, and drinking. When toxic products accumulate or come into the body faster than we expel them, we build up serious health problems.

Various parts of the colon as well as "cleansing" for liver, gall bladder, kidney and so on can be seriously explored. There's ozone water enemas, coffee enemas, and so on — a number of recommended, reliable treatments too numerous to mention here, most requiring professional help, but also many that can be learned from professionals and thereafter safely administered to self.

Many of Sherry Rogers' (M.D.) books will include excellent advice in this area.

Tissue Cleansing Through Bowel Management, by Bernard Jenson, D.C., Ph.D. and Sylvia Bell is also an excellent guide.

Various books on alternative medicine or natural medicine also contain recommendations. Seek them out and work with a health professional on appropriate treatment regimens. You can find the above books, and others, via internet search.

22. What about getting rid of herbicides and pesticides? How do I do it?

One of the fastest and surest means is through the use of a sauna.

The basic purpose of a sauna is to cleanse the body through perspiration. This means opening the pores of the skin and flushing out the impurities in the body through the process of sweating. The sauna of Finland is a tradition which some researchers date back over two thousand years. The Finns attribute their endurance and longevity to the tradition of sauna.

What happens to the body during a sauna is quite simple — your metabolism and pulse rate increases, your blood vessels become much more flexible, and your extremities benefit from increased circulation. Physical fitness fans will recognize that some of these changes can also be achieved through strenuous exercise. Not to say that a sauna would put you in excellent physical condition without moving a muscle, but that it brings about the same metabolic results as physical exercise.

The effects of the sauna are numerous and varied. Proponents of dry heat bath mention a feeling of psychological peace and contentment as well as physical rejuvenation. Many people claim that the sauna relieves the symptoms of minor illnesses such as colds, revives the muscles after tough physical exertion, and clears the complexion. The sauna experience will often leave you feeling very much alive. Your senses will be sharpened, and your tactile sensitivity heightened.

All of the above is accurate and true, and normally refers to short periods of sauna exposure, such as one experiences socially for an hour or two.

L. Ron Hubbard wanted a solution to the drug addiction problem of the sixties and seventies. He found the sauna an important medical answer which was incorporated into the Philosophy of Scientology as a religion.

Zane R. Gard, M.D. was one of the first medical doctors to install a Hubbardian sweat sauna for his medical practice after he, his wife, and daughter were vastly helped from exposure to agent orange. (Go to http://www.arthritistrust.org, "Research" tab, "Research and Letters" tab, and find Zane R. Gard, M.D. in alphabetical list at left of page; Also see "Chemical Exposure" at "Articles Important" tab.)

Oklahoma's Cholocco Indians established a 1000 bed facility utilizing the same process to treat alcoholism and drug addiction, and to teach the proper, effective sauna process. During the interim numerous scientific studies established the great value of Hubbard's sauna technique, and both firemen as well as policemen have benefited through its use from accidental exposure to toxic materials.

Although several medical doctors have made Hubbard's program available for their patients, you should know that every Church of Scientology organization in the world has this process available to you as a "spiritual" program for a cost less than most doctors, and that one does not need to be a Church member to take advantage of it.

Regardless of where you receive this type of sauna, a medical exam is required to assure that your heart can sustain the stress. The program requires consecutive daily attendance for 3-1/2 to 4-1/2 weeks under a temperature of 140 degrees to 180degrees Fahrenheit. You can leave the sauna to cool down for lunch, or a quick shower, if desired, but the idea — as with any sauna — is to sweat copiously over a long period of time.

When sweating, the metabolites and xenobiotics (pesticides and herbicides) that have been stored in the fatty parts of your cells (lipids) mobilize and will start exiting through your sweat pores. These tiny chemical portions are triggering agents for vast responses inside your body that have led to apparent degenerative disease states that have baffled the medical world for generations. For example, you've probably heard of "flashback" caused by the past use of certain illegal drugs, such as LSD. The former LSD user suddenly experiences phenomena as if taking the substances again, when s/he's not actually doing so.

While sweating out these xenobiotic products in the sauna your body/mind/emotions will trigger flashbacks reminding you of operations, sunburn under the beach, drug usage (including prescribed drugs), and so on. These are "triggered" reactions to the activation and expelling of substances previously accumulated in the fatty parts of your cells when your body didn't know what else to do with them.

These xenobiotics (metabolites of pesticides and

herbicides), though minimal in size and well stored in the lipids (fatty cells), are also the source of many poorly understood disease states.

A key element for successful use of the Hubbardian sauna (called the "Purif," or Purification Rundown) is that when the vitamins, minerals and essential fatty acids are sweated out, they're replaced daily by an amount determined by the amount of niacin it requires to produce a flush for that day.

Major differences between the Church of Scientology's sauna and that of medical doctors are that (1) The Church places a partner in the sauna with you who has already been through the experience, and assures that you are experiencing everything OK; and, also the Church has a supervisor review your log of daily events; (2) Unlike the Church, Medical doctors usually take laboratory samples that report on specific xenobiotics and these will be compared against progress in the decrease of your chronic symptoms.

This sauna treatment requires strong will for continued exposure and endurance, but, once you've gone through the initial "want-to-quit" stage, you'll find it easy to endure, and quite beneficial, even restful.

23. After doing all of the above will I be well?

No one knows the answer to such a question!

Keep in mind that you're the camel, and your back is being weighted downward. The key principle to wellness is to began removing the straws that hold you down. How many straws there are, and whether or not you actually remove them is between you and your health professionals. No one — other than you — knows if you've given each straw an honest tug.

Then, too, there may be other straws that we've

not mentioned, or we've not known about. One such, for example, might be problems specific to you such as Diabetes (type II normally can be traced to serious food allergy problems); cancer (a serious systemic and metabolic disease; the tumor is not the cancer!), long-standing metallic poisoning from sources we've not mentioned, and so on. (A former welder got well after decontaminating welding rod metals in his body.)

Of course if you're one of those who've been given a patented drug to alleviate a symptom, and then another to alleviate the side-effects of the first drug, and then another to suppress the side-effects of the second drug — ad infinitum — you've been long-conned into the patented drug game which fattens the portfolio of pharmaceutical company's bottom-line, "health" insurance agents and unthinking doctors! In your drugged state of apathy and slow thought you probably don't have much opportunity to become the lead pack dog to govern your own health.

What to do?

Get away from those *disease* practitioners and find a *health* practitioner!

With some critical exceptions, traditional medical practitioners have an accurate ability to diagnose a medical problem and a lousy ability to cure it. Use their keen ability to diagnose, but seriously question their "solution."

For initial and confirming support of undiagnosed problems you can also take advantage of skilled practitioners of kinesiology and electro-dermal screening. Once accurate diagnosis is assured, you must become the lead pack dog, not your doctor!

Remember, always avoid the authoritarian "Doctor knows best!" approach.

Be honest enough with yourself and the system you use to see palliative treatment for what it is — treatment of a symptom and not a solution for the disease.

Diagnosis and healing remedies should go hand in hand!

And good luck to your straw removal!

Like the happy, standing camel, we pray that you, too, will be full-standing soon!

By the way. If you find a simpler, faster, cheaper way of getting well, please let us know!

24. OK, so I want to get help in the manner you've outlined. Where do I go? How do I find the right kind of health professional?

You've just asked the toughest question! We'll try to answer the best we can at this time.

a. You know your family doctor. Is s/he open-minded? Willing to learn? If yes, then go talk to that person first. We'll be glad to give them free information or references. If not, stay away and search further.

b. Look for doctors who advertise as alternative or complementary or even alternative and general practice. Holistic practitioners may be applicable. Preventive medicine practitioners can be confusing. Many hospitals have jumped on the popular bandwagon for providing "preventive" or "complementary" treatment, but, in fact, have little understanding of the difference between treating causes and treating symptoms. Question the practitioner. Is s/he simply treating your symptoms with herbs instead of drugs? Are they providing some form of "emotional" or "visualization" support, rather than hard, solid curative protocols? (Herbs and other supportive techniques are OK in their place, but, generally, are not solutions to the causes.) After you've absorbed the principles on this website you'll find it easier to distinguish between those who strike for the roots of the disease and those who piddle around its edges.

c. Look on the internet for referral physicians near you. Unfortunately, no one health professional provides all of the medical and dental treatments that may be required for you. Some come close, but regardless of where you live there will most likely be a need to search further for helpful practitioners — several treatments here, several there, and perhaps another far away.

Here are some reputable organizations that can help you find proper physicians or dentists:

To find a biological dentist write or call **The Price-Pottenger Nutrition Foundation**, PO Box 2614, La Mesa, CA 91943-2614; (619) 462-7600.

Or, for a dentist, **American Academy of Biological Dentists**;http//www.biologicaldentistry.org

To find a physician for allergies/chemical sensitivities/addictions **American Academy of Environmental Medicine** call (215) 862-4544)

To find a physician for heart/circulatory problems (chelation therapy) and many other problems write (self-addressed, stamped envelope) **American College for Advancement of Medicine** 23121 Verdugo Dr, Laguna Hills, CA 92653